# Alzheimer's Disease

*Edited by Montasir Elahi*

Published in London, United Kingdom

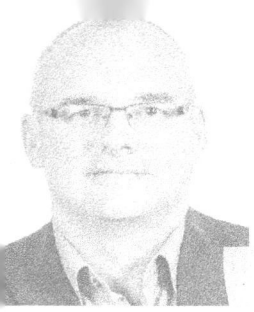
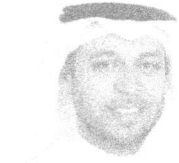
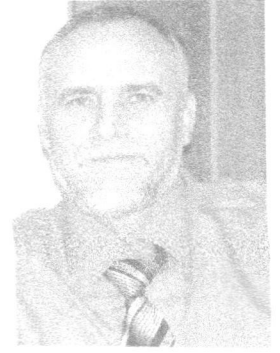
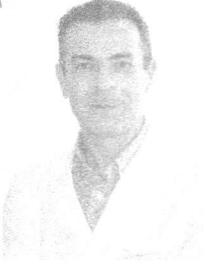
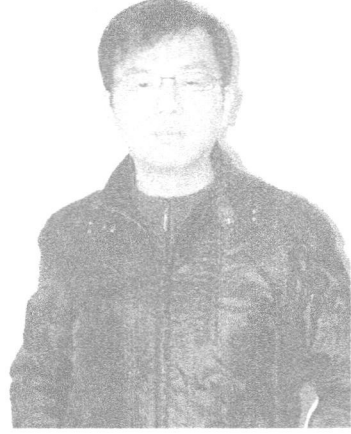
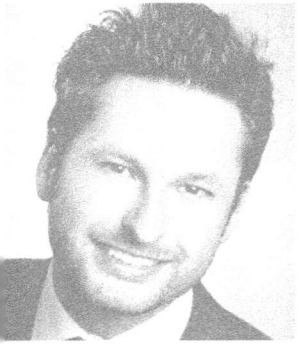
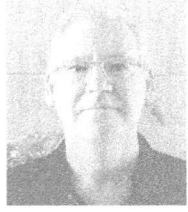

IntechOpen

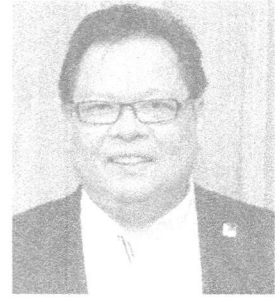
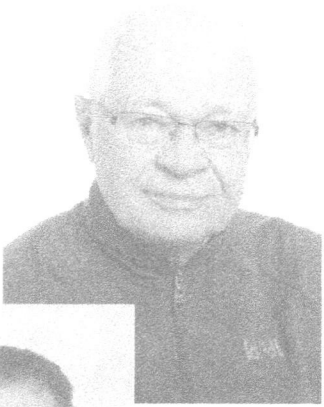
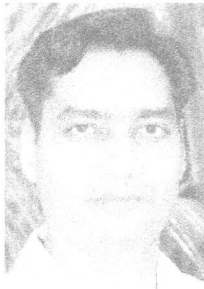
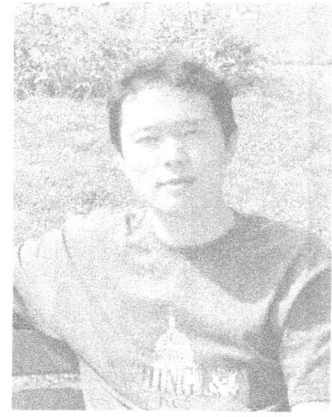
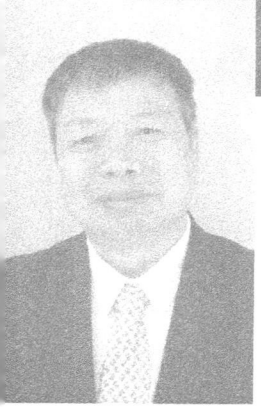
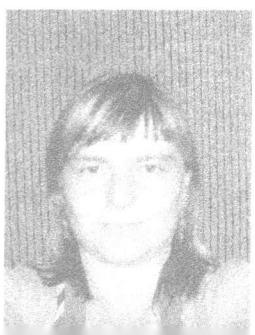

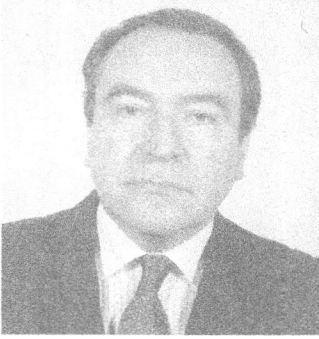

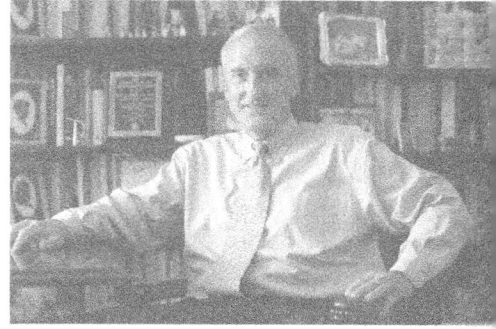

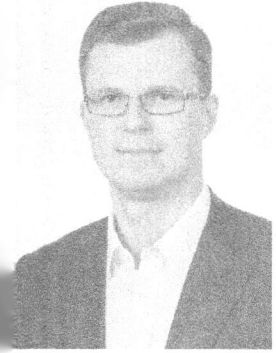

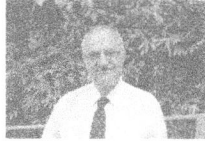

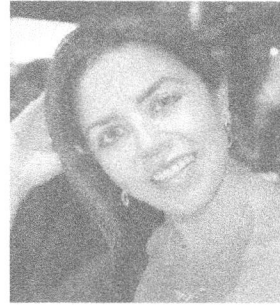

*Supporting open minds since 2005*

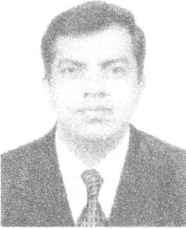

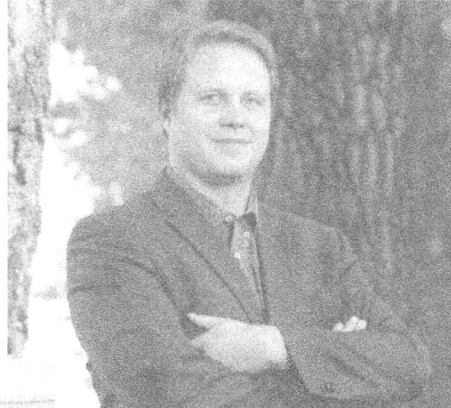

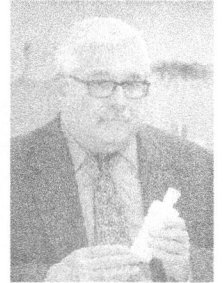

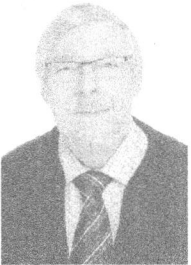

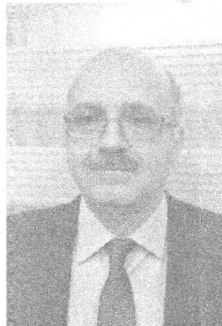

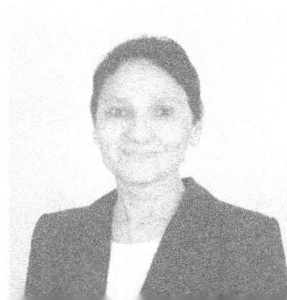

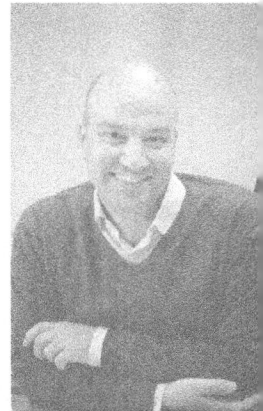

Alzheimer's Disease
http://dx.doi.org/10.5772/intechopen.95246
Edited by Montasir Elahi

Contributors
Afreen Hashmi, Vivek Srivastava, Syed Abul Kalam, Devesh Kumar Mishra, Valentin Bragin, Ilya Bragin, Concetta Crisafulli, Marco Calabrò, Md Alauddin, Afroza Sultana, Bhagawati Saxena, Heena Chauhan, Pawan Gupta

Notice
Statements and opinions expressed in the chapters are these of the individual contributors and not necessarily those of the editors or publisher. No responsibility is accepted for the accuracy of information contained in the published chapters. The publisher assumes no responsibility for any damage or injury to persons or property arising out of the use of any materials, instructions, methods or ideas contained in the book.

First published in London, United Kingdom, 2022 by IntechOpen
IntechOpen is the global imprint of INTECHOPEN LIMITED, registered in England and Wales, registration number: 11086078, 5 Princes Gate Court, London, SW7 2QJ, United Kingdom
Printed in Croatia

British Library Cataloguing-in-Publication Data
A catalogue record for this book is available from the British Library

Additional hard and PDF copies can be obtained from orders@intechopen.com

Alzheimer's Disease
Edited by Montasir Elahi
p. cm.
Print ISBN 978-1-83969-343-4
Online ISBN 978-1-83969-344-1
eBook (PDF) ISBN 978-1-83969-345-8

We are IntechOpen,
the world's leading publisher of
Open Access books
Built by scientists, for scientists

## 6,100+
Open access books available

## 149,000+
International authors and editors

## 185M+
Downloads

Our authors are among the

## 156
Countries delivered to

## Top 1%
most cited scientists

## 12.2%
Contributors from top 500 universities

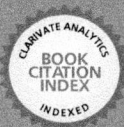

Interested in publishing with us?
Contact book.department@intechopen.com

Numbers displayed above are based on latest data collected.
For more information visit www.intechopen.com

# Meet the editor

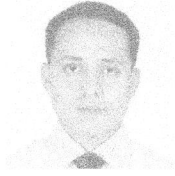

Montasir Elahi currently works as a Research Associate at the University of Maryland, Baltimore, United States of America. He obtained his Bachelor's Degree from the University of Dhaka (Biochemistry and Molecular Biology) in 2003, a Master's Degree from the University of Dhaka in 2004, and a Ph.D. from Tokyo University of Agriculture and Technology (Biotechnology and Life Sciences) in 2014. From 2008 to 2012 he received a Japanese Govt MEXT Fellowship for pursuing doctoral studies. From 2007 to 2008 he worked at the Research Office, International Center for Diarrhoeal Disease Research, Bangladesh. From 2014 to 2016 he was a Post-doctoral fellow at Juntendo University School of Medicine and from 2016 to 2021 he was a Project Assistant Professor at the Department of Diagnosis, Prevention and Treatment of Dementia and Department of Neurology, Juntendo University School of Medicine. Dr. Elahi performs research in Neuroscience, Protein science and Structural biology.

# Contents

# Preface

This Edited Volume is a collection of reviewed and relevant research chapters concerning the recent developments in Alzheimer's disease. The book includes scholarly contributions by various authors and edited by an expert in the field, working on Alzheimer's disease and dementia with cutting-edge technology. Each contribution comes as a separate chapter complete in itself but directly related to the book's topics and objectives.

The book is divided in 5 chapters. The target audience comprises scholars and specialists in the field.

**Montasir Elahi**
University of Maryland,
Baltimore, United States of America

Chapter 1

# Perspective Chapter: Alzheimer - A Complex Genetic Background

*Marco Calabrò and Concetta Crisafulli*

## Abstract

Alzheimer is a complex, multifactorial disease with an ever increasing impact in modern medicine. Research in this area has revealed a lot about the biological and environmental underpinnings of this disease, especially its correlation with B-Amyloid and Tau related mechanics; however, the precise biological pathways behind the disease are yet to be discovered. Recent studies evidenced how several mechanisms, including neuroinflammation, oxidative stress, autophagy failure and energy production impairments in the brain, ---- have been proposed to contribute to this pathology. In this section we will focus on the role of these molecular pathways and their potential link with Alzheimer Disease.

**Keywords:** molecular pathways, genetics, Alzheimer

## 1. Introduction

Alzheimer's disease (AD, MIM: 104300) is the most common neurodegenerative disorder worldwide, accounting for 60% up to 80% of Dementia causes [1]. This disease is one of the fastest rising diseases among the 50 leading causes affecting of life expectancy [2]; according to this trend, the number of AD subjects is destined to rise over 150 million by 2050 [3, 4].

AD worsen with time and as it progresses, patients usually develop short-term to long-term memory loss, accompanied by confusion, irritability and aggression, [5], followed by language impairments and mood swings [6].

Despite its prominence in modern society and the thriving research around it, a lot of its intricate pathophysiology is yet to be discovered. Furthermore, grade and type of symptoms may vary greatly from person to person [7], adding to the complexity of AD. Nevertheless, post mortem observations on AD subjects' Central Nervous System (CNS) evidenced some central histopathological features, mainly focused on amyloid beta (Aβ) plaques and neurofibrillary tangles (NFTs) [8–11].

Aβ plaques are the extracellular deposit of Aβ, which are produced by the cleavage of amyloid precursor protein (APP) [12], while the NFTs consist of abnormal filaments of hyper-phosphorylated Tau by GSK-3β [13]. They are thought to have a significant impact in memory and cognitive function, by triggering synaptic loss or dysfunction and neuronal death [14].

Interestingly, although not all of the causes have been located, AD cases seemingly converge to these hallmarks, providing a steady starting point for trying to understand the biological processes behind this disease.

## 1.1 Genetics

Indeed, among the cases of AD genetic studies individuated a form, known as Familial AD (FAD), that runs in families and is transmitted with an autosomic dominant model [15]. FAD is the best described type of AD: it is associated with mutations in three major genes: APP (chromosome 21), PSEN1 (chromosome 14) and PSEN2 (chromosome 1) [16]. Alterations within these genes affect amyloid

| *Familial AD (FAD)* | OMIM ID |
|---|---|
| An Alzheimer's disease that has_material_basis_in mutation in the gene encoding the amyloid precursor protein on chromosome 21q. | OMIM:104300 |
| An Alzheimer's disease that has_material_basis_in mutation in the presenilin-1 gene (PSEN1) on chromosome 14q24. | OMIM:607822 |
| An Alzheimer's disease that has_material_basis_in a mutation in the presenilin-2 gene (PSEN2) on chromosome 1q42. | OMIM:606889 |
| *Sporadic AD (SAD)* | |
| An Alzheimer's disease that is characterized by an association of the apolipoprotein E E4 allele. | OMIM:104310 |
| An Alzheimer's disease that is characterized by an associated with variation in the region 12p11.23-q13.12. | OMIM:602096 |
| An Alzheimer's disease that is characterized by an associated with variation in the region 10q24. | OMIM:605526 |
| An Alzheimer's disease that is characterized by an associated with variation in the region 10p13. | OMIM:606187 |
| An Alzheimer's disease that is characterized by an associated with variation in the region 20p12.2-q11.21. | OMIM:607116 |
| An Alzheimer's disease that has_material_basis_in heterozygous mutation in ABCA7 on chromosome 19p13.3. | OMIM:608907 |
| An Alzheimer's disease that is characterized by an associated with variation in the region 7q36. | OMIM:609636 |
| An Alzheimer's disease that is characterized by an associated with variation in the region 9p22.1. | OMIM:609790 |
| An Alzheimer's disease that is characterized by an associated with variation in the region 8p12-q22. | OMIM:611073 |
| An Alzheimer's disease that is characterized by an associated with variation in the region 1q21. | OMIM:611152 |
| An Alzheimer's disease that is characterized by an associated with variation in the region 1q25. | OMIM:611154 |
| An Alzheimer's disease that is characterized by an associated with variations in the region 3q22-q24. | OMIM:604154 |
| An Alzheimer's disease that is characterized by an associated with a risk allele in in the PCDH11X gene on chromosome Xq21.3. | OMIM:300756 |
| An Alzheimer's disease that is characterized by an associated with mutations in the gene TREM2. | OMIM:615080 |
| An Alzheimer's disease that has_material_basis_in a mutation in the ADAM10 gene on chromosome 15q21. | OMIM:615590 |
| An Alzheimer's disease that is characterized by associated variants of the gene PLD3. | OMIM:615711 |

**Table 1.**
*Alzheimer sub-types according to genetics [30407550].*

cleavage, directly promoting plaques formation. Several studies demonstrated that alterations in APP or PSEN1 genes are guaranteed to cause AD, while PSEN2 mutations have a 95 percent chance of causing the disease [17]. Unfortunately, only up to 5% of all AD cases are of this type [18].

Other cases usually go under the name of sporadic AD (SAD) which encloses the largest part of AD cases. SAD cases have a more cryptic and heterogenic genetic background [18]: More than 500 candidate genes were correlated with SAD [15, 19, 20]. Of them, inherited polymorphic APOe (chromosome 19) E4 allele is the major risk factor. APOe is the gene encoding for the Apolipoprotein E, whose function is to bind lipids and sterols and transport them through the lymphatic and circulatory systems. APOe4 is thought to produce a more instable form and is related to the formation of neurofibrillary tangles [21, 22] and amyloid clearance processes [23, 24], through a still not well understood mechanism.

### 1.1.1 Apolipoprotein E (APOe)

APOe is in charge of cholesterol transport in the brain [25, 26]. As said before, the e4 isoform of this protein is associated to increased AD-risk [27–30]. The fine molecular mechanisms behind the risk increase operated by APOe4 are not completely characterized, however data obtained from cell cultures evidenced how APOe4 promotes oxidative stress and the generation of neurotoxic fragments which impairs mitochondrial activity [31–33]. In particular, APOe4 isoform seems correlated to an increased α-synuclein (αSyn) accumulation accompanied with synaptic loss, lipid droplet accumulation and dysregulation of intracellular organelles [34]. αSyn is a presynaptic membrane-bound protein abundantly expressed in the brain and is involved in synaptic signaling and membrane trafficking [34]. Further, over other 50 loci/genes have been implicated in SAD [15, 35, 36], underlining AD's complexity and the possibility of it being triggered by different alterations. Indeed, up to date, literature (OMIM and GO) reports 19 different AD subtypes based on different associated loci. **Table 1** reports a summary of such subtypes.

## 2. The pathways of Alzheimer disease

The number of genetic factors described is important contributors to AD. However, neither APOE4 nor the other correlated genes are entirely sufficient to explain (and promote) the totality of AD cases [37].

In such a complex environment represented by multicellular organisms a gene and its product/s is not a stand-alone entity. Each protein interacts with and influences many other elements in a synergic orchestra that regulates an organism.

As such, a single alteration propagates (indirectly) its effects to its interactors following pathways and molecular cascades.

Indeed, rather than single genes, a better approach would be investigating AD as an event related to alterations affecting entire biological pathways. Within this chapter, we will focus on molecular cascades potentially involved in AD. A plethora of mechanisms, including neuroinflammation [38], oxidative stress [39, 40], defects in mitochondrial dynamics and function [41], synaptic and cholinergic malfunctions [42], cholesterol and fatty acid metabolism as well as glucose energetic pathways impairments in the brain [43, 44], autophagy failure [45], apoptosis with multiple cell signaling cascades [42, 46] and other less studied mechanisms have been proposed to contribute to AD. It should be stressed that while they are discussed separately, these pathways are all interlinked and changes in one may very well result in changes in the others.

## 2.1 Hallmarks of AD: Aβ and tau related pathways

Aβ is 4 kDa fragment derived by two subsequent proteolytic cleavages of amyloid precursor protein (APP) by β and γ secretases [47]. As evidenced in studies focused on FAD, genetic alterations of APP, PSEN1 and PSEN2 may negatively influence cleavage promoting Aβ production. Interestingly, contrary to what was once believed, low concentrations of Aβ are seemingly needed to short and long term memory processes [48, 49], and Aβ homeostasis is a lot finer regulated process than once expected, consisting of highly conserved feedback loops and interactions between multiple processes [50].

Potentially risk genes may be found among the ones regulating the biological networks involved in Aβ expression and APP cleavage (including APP, PSEN1, PSEN2, ADAM10, BACE1), its localization and transport (like APOE, CLU, SORL1) and its degradation and clearance (including ABCA7, BIN1, CD2AP, CD33, PICALM, PTK2B and RIN3) [50, 51]. Interestingly, the same elements are interlinked with other important pathways (see later in the text). Aβ accumulation also impairs the structure and function of microglia, astrocytes, and vascular endothelial cells of the brain [52, 53].

The neurotoxic function of Aβ is linked to Tau, a microtubule-associated protein that provides structural assembly and stability of cytoskeletons [54, 55]. The expression of tau is critical during Aβ-mediated synaptotoxic processes where Aβ peptides target phosphorylation-based pathways [55] which hyper-phosphorylate Tau protein through glycogen synthase kinase 3 beta (GSK-3β) and other kinases activated by Aβ peptides [56], and promote their release from microtubules. The removal of Tau from microtubules favors the formation of NFTs composed by aberrantly folded form of hyper-phosphorylated tau and alter the structure of neuritis, giving rise to synaptic malfunction and neuronal death [52].

## 2.2 Oxidative stress

Oxidative stress (OS) has been widely recognized as a prodromal factor associated to AD [57]. According to the current knowledge, increased OS is a sign often observed in the brain of early-stage AD subjects [58]. In particular, OS may act as indicator of changes within the brain. Regarding its correlation with Aβ accumulation, it is known that Aβ is both a cause and the result of OS, as Aβ structure facilitates OS induction [59] and represents a source of radical oxygen and nitrogen species (ROS, RNS) [57]. Through proteic mediators, including NOX, TGF-β, NF-κB and NRF2 genes 'products [60], Aβ increases OS levels and triggers several molecular events that are strictly linked with AD development [61]: OS promotes Tau phosphorylation [62] and also exerts its effect on the choline recycling from the synapse processes, leading to ACh deficiency [63]. It also causes deficit in the energy metabolism (through impairment of mitochondria function and Blood Brain Barrier (BBB) permeability) and leads to apoptosis and then neurodegeneration [64–66]. Of particular relevance, excessive ROS inevitably lead to lipid peroxidation [67], which has been proposed as early biomarker of AD [68]. OS cause damage to all biomolecules. In particular, unsaturated lipids are very sensitive to their action. It should be noted that the brain gray matter and white matter are both very rich in polyunsaturated fatty acids (e.g. docosahexanoic acid, adreinic acid which are brain tissue specific) [69], making the nervous system very sensible to lipid peroxidation [69]. The action of OS in AD through lipid peroxidation is supported by histological evidences showing the co-localization of lipid peroxidation metabolites and Aβ plaques in the brain [70]. Further, it was demonstrated (in culture studies) that the lipids usually found in AD brain lesions produce neurotoxic effects in presence of increased OS levels [71]. Indeed, the chemical reactions following lipid peroxidation often results in the production of isoprostanes and malondialdehyde, which causes DNA damage and toxic stress in cells [72]. Interestingly, the products of lipids peroxidation can be found in bio-fluids such as blood and urines, supporting their potential for diagnosis of AD. As AD potential biomarkers, some of these metabolites were investigated in literature [73]. However, their effective use in clinic is still debated as they showed some promising but contradictory results [68].

## 2.3 Inflammation

Inflammation is a physiological acute event, which is essential to defend the body against toxins and pathogens and for tissue repair. However, if inflammation becomes chronic, it causes detrimental effects with severe consequences. Among the processes involved with AD, the persistent over-activation of the inflammatory cascade represents one of the main biological mechanisms through which AD progresses: indeed, neuroinflammation is not typically associated to AD onset, but it plays a key role in increasing the severity of the disease by exacerbating Aβ and Tau nefarious effects [74–76].

The main players behind cytokines production are the non-neuronal cells that populate the brain, such as microglia, astrocytes, and oligodendrocytes [77–79].

Literature data evidenced that Aβ up-regulates cytokines production by these cells. Further, the presence of Aβ stimulate microglia toward the chronicization of pro-inflammatory state by activating the NF-κB cascade [80–82] or promoting Aβ interaction with FPR2 [83]. Under such conditions, microglia generates a wide range of cytotoxic factors, including interleukins, TNF-α, superoxide, nitric oxide, ROS, prostaglandins and Cathepsin B, which damage extracellular matrix and cause neuronal dysfunction [75, 84]. The increase of cytokines triggers several potentially harmful effects: it induces mitochondrial stress in neurons, either directly or indirectly, including via Aβ signaling. It also increases OS [85, 86] and Blood–Brain Barrier (BBB) permeability which likely influence AD progression [87].

Similar to microglia, astrocytes also produce and/or release an array of inflammatory mediators. Activated or "reactive" astrocytes can be roughly classified in two groups: the "A1" neurotoxic phenotype and the "A2" neuroprotective phenotype based on distinct transcriptional profiles [88]. The A1 group is likely involved with AD through mechanisms similar to microglia.

From a molecular point of view, cytokines like IL-1 and TNF-α promote Aβ production by up-regulating APP and the amyloidogenic secretases [81, 89], while IL-6 and IL-18 promote Tau hyper-phosphorylation [90, 91].

Ultimately, a cycle is established in which inflammation increases Aβ production (and triggers other negative processes increasing protein accumulation and OS), which in turn stimulate microglia to maintain its pro-inflammatory state. The uncontrolled cytokines production then causes neuronal death [38] as it damages synapses (please refer to Section 2.4), myelin sheaths and axons, promote complement-mediated damage and/or triggers apoptotic or necroptotic mechanisms [92]. This link between AD and microglia is also supported by Genome wide association studies, which evidenced how several genes (TREM2, CLU, CR1, EPHA1, ABCA7, MS4A4A/MS4A6E, CD33, CD2AP) related with an increased AD risk regulate glial inflammatory reaction [75]. Additionally, it has been observed that astrocyte-based inflammatory cascade could recruit peripheral macrophages, white blood cells, and lymphocytes that infiltrate brain parenchyma thanks to BBB increased permeability and vascular alterations [93].

## 2.4 Neurodevelopment and neurotransmission associated processes

Neurodevelopmental/Neuroplasticity and Neurotransmission related pathways are likely associated with AD development and in particular with its cognitive symptoms [94]. Physiologically, these processes consist in the proliferation, differentiation and maturation of neural stem cells (NSC) and the modulation of their interactions through synapse- and neurotransmission- related processes.

Regarding neurodevelopment processes, it has been observed that the synaptic pruning pathway becomes aberrantly up regulated in the first stages of AD. This aberrant activation, which leads to synaptic loss [95], seems to be triggered by Aβ, through PANX1, ryanodine receptor (RyR) function [96, 97] other than several inflammatory signals [98].

PANX1 is a protein involved in the modulation of neurotransmission, neurogenesis and synaptic plasticity [99]. An increase of this protein under inflammatory conditions contributes to neuronal death [100].

RyR is Ca2+ channel which modulates different processes including neuronal development and plasticity [101].

The anomalous RyR channel function is triggered by Aβ and OS through Ca2+ increased concentrations [96] and are interlinked to mitochondrial and NOX2-mediated ROS generation [102] and glial activation [103].

Regarding the inflammatory elements, it has been observed that many cytokines directly interact with receptors located on neuronal membranes. Here they activate or modulate pathways involved in synaptic function and plasticity (e.g. p38 MAPK and NFκB pathways). Further, synapse function and stability are also heavily regulated by microglia and astrocytes. In particular, the former is seemingly implicated in pruning mechanics [95], while the latter appear to have an heavy involvement in regulating synapse formation, stability, and turnover [104]. Astrocytes physically wrap synapses. The synapse/astrocyte interface is fairly active as astrocytes release numerous proteins capable of modulating synaptic function, sprouting and remodeling.

Regarding neurotransmission, several reports have indicated a significant reduction of Serotonin (5-HT) [105], Dopamine (DA) [106] and Norepinephrine (NE) [107] levels as well as their receptors in AD brain. In AD, loss of 5-HT results in depression, anxiety and agitation [108], dysregulation of DA release leads to reward-mediated memory formation deficits [109] and low level of NE impairs spatial memory function [110]. Glutamatergic and cholinergic abnormalities in particular, were pointed as one of the principal causes of cognitive deterioration in AD.

### 2.4.1 Cholinergic neurotransmission

The cholinergic system regulates attention processing [111], cognition [111], memory function and behavior via the release of the neurotransmitter acetylcholine (ACh) [112].

Several studies evidenced how ACh production and reuptake are impaired in AD brains [113]. Further, accumulation of intraneuronal Aβ degenerates basal forebrain cholinergic neurons and reduces ACh levels [114], which in turn leads to memory deficits [115]. A potential candidate through which Aβ exerts its effect is α7nAChRs. Studies on α7nAChRs KO models evidenced how the lack of this receptor could induce AD-like pathology, including Aβ increase. In addition, its depletion is linked to an increased age-dependent expression of phosphorylated Tau [116, 117].

About the mechanisms underlying α7nAChR regulation of Aβ production, it seems that physiologically this receptor activations shifts APP processing toward the non-amyloidogenic pathway [118], enhancing the production of the neuro-protective APPα (soluble form) which is able to counteract Aβ neurotoxicity [119]. Interestingly, α7nAChRs mediate the intake of pre-synaptic Ca2+ levels during neuronal activity, indirectly modulating all biological processes dependent on this ion, glutamate release, synaptic transmission, and cognitive function [120]. When α7nAChRs is reduced, a negative feedback mechanism is triggered which increase Aβ production with the aim of maintaining Ca2+ influx in the cells [121]. Aβ in turn, further decrease its expression. This reduction ultimately exerts its effect on the N-methyl-D-aspartate receptor (NMDAR), which is removed from membrane, and on nicotinic and MAPK signaling, resulting in the development of cognitive deficits [122].

### 2.4.2 Glutamatergic neurotransmission

The most common excitatory neurotransmitter, glutamate, and its receptors are required for neuronal cell differentiation, migration, survival, and synaptic plasticity. There are two types of glutamate receptors: ionotropic glutamate receptors (iGluRs), such as N-methyl-D-aspartate (NMDA), α-Ammino-3-idrossi-5-Metil-4-isossazol-Propionic Acid (AMPA) and Kainate receptors; and metabotropic glutamate receptors (mGluRs).

Over-activation of these receptors causes neuronal excitotoxicity as well as neuronal death, and this is thought to be one of the mechanism causing neurodegeneration in AD [123]. Indeed, in patients with AD, available evidence points to a disruption in the glutamatergic neurotransmission cycle at the point of glial cell reuptake of free glutamate from the synapse: Aβ can interfere with glutamate receptors and transporters [96]. The binding of such receptors triggers neuronal susceptibility to glutamate excitotoxicity, dyshomeostasis and defective plasticity [124]. The biological mechanism is still not well understood, but likely needs the function of a tyrosine-protein kinase, Fyn, which alter NMDARs function through phosphorylation [125]. Interestingly, Astrocytes may also play a role in the impaired glutamate clearance from the synaptic cleft. As said before, astrocytes wrap synapses. In the synaptic interface, these cells present a high concentration of excitatory amino acid transporters (EAATs), including EAAT1 and EAAT2. Physiologically, over 80% of extracellular glutamate is taken by astrocytes through these transportes [126]. It has been observed that Aβ peptides and pro-inflammatory elements down regulate the expression of EAATs, impairing glutamate clearance [127]. As such, free glutamate accumulates out of synapses while the vesicular glutamate uptake is reduced. The consequence of this condition is a chronic low-level activation of glutamatergic receptors on postsynaptic neurons and reduced sensibility to glutamate during neuronal firing (due to the low concentration of the neurotransmitter within vesicles) [128], leading to suboptimal neurotransmission and impairment of long-term potentiation (LTP) [128].

## 2.5 Energy metabolism

Energy is of high importance to maintain the physiological function of the brain. Processes related to energy production (Glucose intake, ATP production) are disrupted in AD brains [129]: Indeed, several brain areas in AD patients show a significant decrease of glucose metabolism [130]. Additionally, the first AD-related intracellular lesions usually develop in neurons with a higher energy consumption [131] and often involve enzymes related to tricarboxylic acid cycle, which lead neurons to a hypo-metabolic state [63].

Interestingly, an excess of an important energy substrate, glucose, may also lead to the exacerbation of AD symptomatology. A high glucose concentration is also the main characteristic of diabetes. Other than being a risk factor for the development of diabetic complications, it seems to play a role in the development of AD cognitive symptoms [132].

Indeed, high levels of glucose are harmful for the brain, as they lead to Aβ accumulation on brain lesions. It also exacerbates OS and promotes neuroinflammation [133, 134], with the consequences already described in the previous sections.

Glucose levels are affected by numerous elements, such as pro-inflammatory cytokines [135, 136]. However, the main control is exerted by the antagonistic function of insulin and glucagon.

Insulin signaling has been the focus of multiple AD studies [137–139] were it was shown that both Aβ deposition and tau hyperphosphorylation are correlated with the impairment of Insulin signaling cascade [140, 141], and insulin resistance in particular.

According to these observations, insulin resistance is a feature of both type 2 diabetes mellitus (T2DM) and AD, supporting a biological overlapping between the two pathologies. As said before, the high glucose condition increases Aβ production. On a molecular level this increase is linked to the inhibition of APP degradation pathways [142].

Chronic hyperinsulinemia in brain also leads to cognitive dysfunctions [143], Insulin receptor is present in hippocampus [144], the main area responsible for memory. A chronic exposition to insulin favors a resistance mechanism, making neurons less responsive to this hormone. Further, Aβ can interact with insulin receptors causing their internalization and thus inhibiting their function [145]. Additionally, Aβ seizing insulin receptor, increases insulin levels in the brain microenvironment, which in turn promote inflammation increasing TNFα, interleukin 1β and 6 (IL1β and IL6) [146].

Through a still not completely understood mechanic, the alteration of insulin signaling (or an increased resistance to insulin) ultimately triggers neuroinflammation and neurodegeneration, increasing Aβ concentrations and Tau hyperphosphorylation [145, 147].

## 2.6 Autophagy impairments

Autophagy is an intracellular process mediated by vesicles and lysosomes that consists of several sequential steps which ultimately lead to the degradation of damaged/misfolded proteins and dysfunctional organelles, thereby sustaining cellular homeostasis [148].

Physiologically, this process is especially important for neuronal and glial cells health [149, 150]. Although it is still not clear whether dysfunction of autophagy is the cause or result of AD [151], it has been observed that the dysregulation of autophagy may occur in early stage of the disease. In particular, this process is believed to be a major pathway for Aβ clearance/accumulation [152] and is also involved in the pathological mechanisms of neurodegeneration [149, 150]. Studies on animal models also reported that restoring the physiological autophagosomes clearance ameliorate/prevents AD cognitive symptoms [153].

Studies on AD brains revealed a significantly higher presence of autophagosomal and pre-lysosomal vacuoles in neuronal dendrites and axons [154–156]. These vacuoles were shown to be enriched in APP, γ-secretase components, PSEN1 and nicastrin, which are required to generate Aβ [157, 158]. According to the autophagic hypothesis, the block of autophagy and the consequent accumulation of autophagosomes trigger neuronal degeneration [156] and leads to the release of these vesicles in the extracellular space where they form the characteristic AD plaques [159, 160]. Autophagy is also essential for Tau clearance [161]. Usually, Tau is transported in vacuole for degradation, however certain mutations of Tau, cause the block of this protein in the membrane of lysosome. The accumulation in the membrane impairs and disrupts lysosomes function and structure, which ultimately lead to the release of lysosomal enzymes in the cytoplasm [161].

Recent studies have proven that autophagy could be influenced by diverse factors, such as Aβ [162] and OS [163]. In addition, ApoE4 and Aβ influence of lysosomal membranes stability [164].

From a biological point of view, autophagy is mainly regulated according to the physiological condition of cells through several elements:

*ATG7* is a key gene regulating autophagy process [150]. It is involved in degradation of tau [165] and mediates the transport of Aβ peptides [166]. Alterations of its function have been correlated with AD [167].

Beclin 1 (*BECN1/ATG6*) protein mediates the initiation of autophagy [150]. BECN1 is involved in the pathophysiology of AD. The expression of BECN1 is decreased in brains of AD patients when compared with healthy individuals [168]. Decreasing of Becn1 expression leads to increased levels of Aβ [168] and also increases microglia inflammatory response [169].

The down-regulation of this protein is believed to be caused by caspase-3 up-regulation [170]. Further, BCL2 Apoptosis Regulator (BCL2) is an anti-apoptotic factor that regulate autophagy through BECN1 [171]. The overexpression of Bcl2 has protective effects against Aβ-driven neuronal death [170]. The overexpression of Bcl2 affects also tau processing, reducing the number of NFTs [170].

Cyclin Dependent Kinase 5 (CDK5) is an autophagy-regulating kinase [150], which influences the metabolism and effects of Aβ. CDK5 likely act through regulation of β-secretase, which is a crucial enzyme involved in APP metabolism [172]. This kinase also mediates Aβ peptide-induced dendritic spine loss [173], providing a pathway linking Aβ with cognitive dysfunction. Similarly, CDK5 is similarly involved in tau phosphorylation [174], although it seems to not be sufficient to trigger NFT formation [174].

Clusterin (*CLU/APOJ*) is a chaperone protein implicated in autophagosomes biogenesis via interaction with ATG8E (MAP1LC3A) [150]. According to meta-analyses data on AD subjects, *this protein is* one of the top AD candidate genes [37, 175, 176]. Its alterations have been suggested to affect neuron connectivity in several brain regions [177, 178]. Physiologically, CLU interacts with Aβ, preventing its aggregation [179, 180].

Cathepsin D (*CTSD*) is a lysosomal protease [150] involved in APP and Aβ degradation [181]. Its role and correlation in AD is still under debate as literature produced controversial results [182–185].

Alpha-Synuclein (*SNCA/PARK1/NACP*) is another protein found to be associated with AD risk [150]. SNCA is an important component of Aβ plaques [186] and can influence the expression of/be regulated by Aβ peptides [187, 188]. Similarly, to interaction of SNCA with Aβ peptides, SNCA and tau also induce each other fibrilization [189]. SNCA binds, phosphorylates, and inhibits microtubule assembly activity of tau [190].

PINK1 and PRKN genes products are important elements behind autophagosome-mediated mitochondrial degradation [191]. In AD, high levels of Aβ inhibit the expression of those proteins, leading to increased dysfunctional lysosomes and neurodegeneration [192, 193].

Ubiquilin 1 (*UBQLN1*) is involved in autophagosome–lysosome fusion [150], likely through ATG8E (MAP1LC3A) [194]. Meta-analyses *studies correlate UBQLN1* with an increased risk for AD [195, 196]. It has been observed that the expression of UBQLN1 is reduced in AD patients [197, 198]. This decrease, in turn, up-regulates APP processing [198].

Ubiquitin C-Terminal Hydrolase L1 (*UCHL1*) influences autophagy by interaction with LAMP2 which modulates autophagosome-lysosome fusion [150]. Uchl1 interacts with App [199]. Its over expression decreases Aβ and NFT production [199] and lower levels of UCHL1 have been found in AD patients [200]. Regarding its autophagic role, it has been observed that UCHL1 is involved in lysosomal degradation of BACE1 [200].

Of all the described autophagic regulators potentially linked with AD, the mammalian target of rapamycin (mTOR) has been studied most investigated and is considered to play a key role in autophagy biogenesis. The mTOR protein acts as inhibitor in autophagy regulation through different pathways, including AMPK and PI3-Akt [201, 202]. In neurons and glial cells, mTOR is highly expressed an play an important role for synaptic plasticity and memory [202]. In neurons and glial cells, mTOR proteins are highly expressed, and their modulatory activities are fundamental in brain development. In the adult brain, mTOR signaling plays a crucial role in the translational initiation of protein synthesis required for synaptic plasticity and memory formation. However, uncontrolled mTOR activity leads to impairment of such processes. Numerous studies on AD brains and AD mice models revealed mTOR hyper-activation in AD brain [203]: Aβ accumulation seems to promote the activation mTOR pathway through phosphorylation of the mTOR inhibitor PRAS40 [204]. Further, hypo-energetic states may also activate mTOR [146].

Interestingly, a defective autophagy in other cells, including Astrocytes, microglia, and oligodendrocytes has also been linked to AD. In particular, disturbing basal autophagy processes in glia trigger neuroinflammation, which, as previously described, is an important pathway leading to the progression of AD [205].

## 2.7 Cerebrovascular abnormalities

In patients with AD, cerebrovascular abnormalities are a common comorbidity [206, 207]. These may contribute to the onset of cognitive impairment and dementia. Altered cerebral blood flow and pressure at the level of the brain are induced vascular dysfunction [208]. These events are injurious to normal brain function that would result in disturbed homeostasis, but also in blood–brain barrier (BBB) damage and micro-fractures in cerebral vases [209]. It has also been observed that the permeability of BBB to immune cells and molecules increases with aging. As said in the previous sections, the infiltration of immune cells in the brain parenchyma favors neuroinflammation [210] and ROS production [206], thus increasing the risk of AD [81].

These events are linked to the formation of Aβ plaques [211]. In particular, ROS production is related to the increase of the Advanced Glycation Endproducts (AGE) proteins and their receptors (RAGE) in the vascular system [212, 213]. A chronic hypo-perfusion state favors the formation of Aβ through the activation of the adaptive response to hypoxia and reduced clearance via perivascular draining [214, 215]. Furthermore, Aβ accumulation seems to be mainly localized in brain areas with reduced cerebral blood flow [216]. Finally, as said before, AD brains are in a pro-inflammatory state; in these conditions Notch signaling is up regulated [217]. Notch signaling has an essential role in vascular development and angiogenesis in brain through the modulation of VEGFR2 [218]. It has been observed that chronic activation of Notch1 negatively affect the brain microenvironment, in particular the delicate connection of the brain with cardiovascular system. Indeed, Notch signaling, in association with VEGF, has been demonstrated to cause impaired blood flow, further reducing the nutrients intake by neurons (worsening the already weak energetic state). Notch also induces BBB leakages, which has severe impact on the brain and may accelerate Aβ accumulation [217]. BBB homeostasis also depends on the role of astrocytes as the act as bridge between the vascular and neuronal compartment. Several studies have observed that astrocytes go through morphological changes in proximity of vascular Aβ deposits [219]. These alterations likely occur during early stages of the disease and evidence a neurovascular uncoupling, which ultimately lead to a dysfunction of BBB barrier. It has been observed that the alteration of astrocytes induces an age-dependent accumulation of amyloid [220].

### 2.8 Signal transduction

#### 2.8.1 Alteration in PKC signaling

Protein kinase C (PKC) family in mammalian is divided in three subfamily: a) calcium-dependent PKC (cPKC), necessity of DAG and $Ca^{2+}$ presence for triggering; b) calcium-independent isoforms (nPKC), that requires DAG presence; c) an atypical isoform of PKC (aPKC) [221]. PKC isoforms are involved in several neural processes, including the ones related to cognitive function. The cPKC and nPKC isoforms could have impact on synaptic formation and plasticity, spatial memory organization or dendritic loss [221], while aPKC isoform is involved in long-term memory [222]. A deficiency in PKC isoforms signaling is thought to be involved in AD [223]. Indeed, deficiency of bPKC is correlated with Tau hyper-phosphorylation (through GSK-3b) while lack cPKC and nPKC activation down-regulates α-secretase activity [222, 224]. Furthermore, Aβ contributes to inhibit PKC isozymes [223, 224].

#### 2.8.2 Wnt signaling pathway

The Wnt signaling pathways play a crucial role in the central nervous system during all phases of neuronal growth and development and remain significant in the adult nervous system [225]. In adults, this process is particularly important since it manages memory creation, maintenance, and behavior. Alteration of this process is strongly linked to neurodegeneration [225]. Altered function of Wnt signaling components was detected in AD brain, including down regulation of b-catenin translocation into the nucleus [226]. The reduction of b-catenin in neurons nuclei triggers the overexpression of the Wnt antagonist GSK-3b and Dkk-1 [225, 227]. GSK-3b, as discussed before, is the main enzyme in charge of tau hyperphosphorylation. Furthermore, it participates in OS generation, which ultimately disrupts neuronal function [227].

#### 2.8.3 Calcium role

Cellular $Ca^{2+}$ is a key ion involved in the regulation several processes in neurons [228, 229]. Its dyshomeostasis may play a key role in the pathogenesis of AD [230] and may even precede the formation of Aβ plaques and NFTs [228].

Intracellular $Ca^{2+}$ is usually stored in the Endoplasmatic Reticulum. Its release in the cytosol is finely controlled by multiple pathways, including RyRs and inositol 1,4,5-trisphosphate receptors (InsP3R) -related ones [231]. Even its intake from the extracellular environment is tightly regulated by multiple processes, such as the store-operated Ca2+ entry (SOCE) pathway and the voltage-gated $Ca^{2+}$ channels (VGCC) [232].

As discussed before in the neurotransmission section, the physiological $Ca^{2+}$ influx stimulates the processing of APP by α-secretase [230], thus protecting from Aβ accumulation. Imbalanced cellular $Ca^{2+}$ contributes to pathophysiological conditions such as accumulation of Aβ plaques and neurofibrillary tangles, protein misfolding, necrosis, apoptosis, autophagy deficits, and degeneration [230, 233].

Finally, excess cytosolic $Ca^{2+}$ concur in mitochondria dysfunction and dysregulates KIF5-Miro-Trak-mediated mitochondrial transport to synapses [63].

High OS states and the presence of Aβ can interfere with $Ca^{2+}$ homeostasis, releasing it from ER stores through the InsP3R and RyR [230, 234]. In addition, the increased intracellular $Ca^{2+}$ levels in the cells interfere with the physiological function of VGCCs, thus impairing neurotransmission [230, 233].

### 2.9 Balance of phosphorylation: Kinases and phosphatases

Protein phosphorylation and dephosphorylation are two essential cellular mechanisms through which a wide-range of receptors and trasduction cascades are regulated. Numerous kinases and phosphatases are encoded in our genome; these two class of enzymes works balancing each other, maintaining an equilibrium phosphorylation and dephosphorylation. Impairment of such finely regulated process has been correlated with AD. As said before in this chapter, one of the trademarks of AD is the hyperphosphorylation of Tau protein, which triggers in a prion-like manner the formation of NFTs. It has been observed that Tau protein has over 85 potential phosphorylation sites [235].

There are several protein kinases that could phosphorylate Tau [236], some of them involved in the pathways discussed so far, including gsk-3β, cdk5, microtubule affinity regulated kinases (mark), tau-tubulin kinases (ttbk), Tyrosine-protein kinase Fyn (Fyn) or Tyrosine-protein kinase Abl1 (Abl1), protein kinase A (pka), Calcium/calmodulin-dependent protein kinase (CaMKII) [236, 237]. All of these kinases have been correlated with an increased risk of AD and are capable of phosphorylate tau at multiple sites [237]. In particular, it appears that phosphorylation of Thr231 and Ser262 residues are critical for NFTs formation.

Hyperphosphorylation of Tau can also be reached and maintained through inhibition of phosphatases. Protein phosphatase 2A (PP2A) is the major enzyme that accounts for ~71% of the total tau dephosphorylation activity [238]. This enzyme co-localizes with tau and microtubules in the brain [239]. In AD, the activity of PP2A is decreased [240]. Interestingly, its down-regulation not only decrease the dephosphorylating activity but also activates CaM-KII and PKA pathways, favoring hyperphosphorylation, as it has been observed in some in vitro and in vivo studies [241, 242].

Other phosphatases have also a role in AD, including Striatal-Enriched protein tyrosine Phosphatase is an intracellular phosphatase (STEP), protein phosphatase 1 (PP1), protein phosphatase 5 (PP5), Calcineurin (PP2B), PP2C [243], through complex feedback mechanisms.

In particular, recent evidences pointed to STEP as one of the targets via which Aβ exerts its deleterious effects in AD. Elevated levels of Aβ seems to be involved in the activation of Step through the activation of α7nAChRs [244, 245] and the subsequent increase of calcium influx [245]. This triggers a cascade of molecular events (in which PP2B and PP1 are also involved) that ultimately activate STEP. STEP mediates the Aβ-induced cognitive impairment by dephosphorylation of important elements involved in synaptic plasticity and dendritic density (such as SPIN90, PSD-95 and Shank), eventually causing the collapse of synapses [246, 247].

Interestingly, the regulation of kinases and phosphatases is strictly linked to glucose metabolism, through the protein kinase AMPK (Ampk). Moreover, Aβ transiently inhibit AMPK potentially providing a link between Aβ and metabolic defects in the AD brain [248]. The activation of AMPK is correlated with glucose metabolism and is related to gluconeogenesis, IR and insulin deficiency. AMPK mediates phosphorylation and signal transduction through GSK-3β [249], PP2A [250], beta-secretase 1 (BACE1) and sirtuin1 (SIRT1). In addition, through SIRT1, AMPK promotes autophagy. Physiologically AMPK cascade inhibits hyperphosphorylation of tau and can reduce Aβ production. Impairments of this cascade potentially lead to AD progression.

## 3. Conclusions

AD is one of the main causes of disability and decreased quality of life world-wide. Despite the ever-increasing number of studies, many fundamental questions remain regarding the molecular background of this disease.

The evidences derived from the recent data on AD stress its "multifactorial nature" and clearly indicate the necessity to consider wider approaches while trying to understand its biological mechanics. This chapter wanted to contribute toward and stress this new 'pathway-like' perspective on AD. A much deeper discussion would be needed to explore the cascades potentially linked with the disease and surely, a lot is still to be discovered. Research activity in this area is very fervid a new data is accumulating daily in the scientific community. As a final but very important note, our genes and pathways (altered or not) do respond, interacts and adapt 'continuously' to external stimuli. Although they were not discussed here, these environmental factors should always be considered as they can greatly influence the biological mechanisms behind multifactorial pathologies such as AD [1, 251]. Further, Epigenetic dysregulation also seems to be involved in AD as methylation mechanics [252, 253] and miRNAs signaling [254] have been found to be altered in AD brain. The key to further deepen the studies of AD would be to understand how all these processes interact and influence with each other and act in concert toward this disease progression.

## Conflict of interest

The authors declare no conflict of interest.

## Notes/thanks/other declarations

We want to thank all of the scientific community and people who spend their effort for the progress of our knowledge.

## Nomenclature

| | |
|---|---|
| 5-HT | Serotonin |
| ABCA7 | ATP Binding Cassette Subfamily A Member 7 |
| ACh | Acetylcholine |
| AD | Alzheimer's disease |
| ADAM10 | ADAM Metallopeptidase Domain 10 |
| AGE | Advanced Glycation Endproducts |
| AMPA | α-Ammino-3-idrossi-5-Metil-4-isossazol-Propionic Acid |
| AMPK | 5′ adenosine monophosphate-activated protein kinase |
| aPKC | atypical isoform of PKC |
| APOe | Apolipoprotein E gene |

APP             Amyloid precursor protein
Aβ              Amyloid beta
BACE1           Beta-Secretase 1
BBB             Blood Brain Barrier
BIN1            Bridging Integrator 1
CD2AP           CD2 Associated Protein
CD33            CD33 Molecule
CLU             Clusterin
CNS             Central Nervous System
cPKC            calcium-dipendent PKC
DA              Dopamine
DAG             diacylglycerol
DKK1            Dickkopf-1
ER              Endoplasmatic Reticulum
FAD             Familiar AD
FPR2            formyl peptide receptor type 2
GBA
GSK-3b          glycogen synthase kinase 3 beta
iGluRs          Ionotropic glutamate receptors
IL-1            Interleukin-1
IL-18           Interleukin-18
IL1β            interleukin 1β
IL-6            Interleukin-6
InsP3R          inositol 1,4,5-trisphosphate receptors
KIF5a           kinesin family member 5a
LTP             long-term potentiation
MAPK            mitogen-activated protein kinase
mGluRs          metabotropic glutamate receptors
Miro            mitochondrial Rho GTPases
mTOR            Mammalian target of rapamycin
NE              Norepinephrine
NFTs            neurofibrillary tangles
NF-κB           nuclear factor kappa light chain enhancer of activated B cells
NMDA            N-methyl-D-aspartate
NMDAR           N-methyl-D-aspartate receptor
NOX             NADPH oxidase
NOX2            NADPH oxidase-2
nPKC            calcium-indipendent PKC
Nrf2            nuclear factor erythroid 2–related factor 2
NSC             neural stem cells
OS              Oxidative Stress
PANX1           Pannexin 1
PI3-Akt         phosphoinositide-3-kinase - protein kinase B
PICALM          Phosphatidylinositol Binding Clathrin Assembly Protein
PINK1           PTEN-induced kinase 1
PKC             Protein kinase C
PRAS40          AKT1 Substrate 1
PSEN1           presenilin-1
PSEN2           presenilin-2
PTK2B           Protein Tyrosine Kinase 2 Beta
RAGE            Advanced Glycation Endproducts Receptors
RIN3            Ras And Rab Interactor 3
RNS             Radical nitrogen species

| ROS | Radical oxygen species |
| RyR | ryanodine receptor |
| SAD | sporadic AD |
| SOCE | store-operated Ca2+ entry |
| SORL1 | Sortilin Related Receptor 1 |
| TGF β | Transforming Growth Factor-β |
| TNF-α | Tumor necrosis factor α |
| Trak1 | trafficking kinesin protein 1 |
| VEGF | Vascular-Endothelial Growth Factor |
| VEGFR2 | Vascular endothelial growth factor receptor 2 |
| VGCC | voltage-gated Ca2+ channels |
| Wnt | Wingless-related integration site |
| α7nAChRs | α7 nicotinic acetylcholine receptor |
| αSyn | α-synuclein |

## Author details

Marco Calabrò and Concetta Crisafulli*
Department of Biomedical and Dental Sciences and Morphofunctional Imaging,
University of Messina, Italy

*Address all correspondence to: ccrisafulli@unime.it

IntechOpen

## References

[1] Alzheimer's Association. 2020 Alzheimer's disease facts and figures. Alzheimer's & dementia: The Journal of the Alzheimer's Association. 2020;**16**:391-460

[2] Kumar A, Sidhu J, Goyal A, Tsao JW. Alzheimer Disease. Treasure Island (FL): StatPearls; 2021

[3] da Silva AP, Chiari LPA, Guimaraes AR, Honorio KM, da Silva ABF. Drug design of new 5-HT6R antagonists aided by artificial neural networks. Journal of Molecular Graphics & Modelling. 2021;**104**:107844

[4] Eguchi K, Shindo T, Ito K, Ogata T, Kurosawa R, Kagaya Y, et al. Whole-brain low-intensity pulsed ultrasound therapy markedly improves cognitive dysfunctions in mouse models of dementia - Crucial roles of endothelial nitric oxide synthase. Brain Stimulation. 2018;**11**(5):959-973

[5] Reisberg B, Borenstein J, Salob SP, Ferris SH, Franssen E, Georgotas A. Behavioral symptoms in Alzheimer's disease: Phenomenology and treatment. The Journal of Clinical Psychiatry. 1987;**48**(Suppl):9-15

[6] Klimova B, Maresova P, Valis M, Hort J, Kuca K. Alzheimer's disease and language impairments: social intervention and medical treatment. Clinical Interventions in Aging. 2015;**10**:1401-1407

[7] Lam B, Masellis M, Freedman M, Stuss DT, Black SE. Clinical, imaging, and pathological heterogeneity of the Alzheimer's disease syndrome. Alzheimer's Research & Therapy. 2013;**5**(1):1

[8] Jack CR Jr, Albert MS, Knopman DS, McKhann GM, Sperling RA, Carrillo MC, et al. Introduction to the recommendations from the National Institute on Aging-Alzheimer's Association workgroups on diagnostic guidelines for Alzheimer's disease. Alzheimer's & Dementia: The Journal of the Alzheimer's Association. 2011; 7(3):257-262

[9] Albert MS, DeKosky ST, Dickson D, Dubois B, Feldman HH, Fox NC, et al. The diagnosis of mild cognitive impairment due to Alzheimer's disease: Recommendations from the National Institute on Aging-Alzheimer's Association workgroups on diagnostic guidelines for Alzheimer's disease. Alzheimer's & Dementia: The Journal of the Alzheimer's Association. 2011;7(3): 270-279

[10] McKhann GM, Knopman DS, Chertkow H, Hyman BT, Jack CR Jr, Kawas CH, et al. The diagnosis of dementia due to Alzheimer's disease: recommendations from the National Institute on Aging-Alzheimer's Association workgroups on diagnostic guidelines for Alzheimer's disease. Alzheimer's & Dementia: The Journal of the Alzheimer's Association. 2011; 7(3):263-269

[11] Yang EJ, Mahmood U, Kim H, Choi M, Choi Y, Lee JP, et al. Phloroglucinol ameliorates cognitive impairments by reducing the amyloid beta peptide burden and pro-inflammatory cytokines in the hippocampus of 5XFAD mice. Free Radical Biology & Medicine. 2018; **126**:221-234

[12] Tanzi RE, Gusella JF, Watkins PC, Bruns GA, St George-Hyslop P, Van Keuren ML, et al. Amyloid beta protein gene: cDNA, mRNA distribution, and genetic linkage near the Alzheimer locus. Science. 1987;**235**(4791):880-884

[13] Mandelkow EM, Mandelkow E. Tau in Alzheimer's disease. Trends in Cell Biology. 1998;**8**(11):425-427

[14] Marsh J, Alifragis P. Synaptic dysfunction in Alzheimer's disease: The effects of amyloid beta on synaptic vesicle dynamics as a novel target for therapeutic intervention. Neural Regeneration Research. 2018;**13**(4): 616-623

[15] Calabro M, Rinaldi C, Santoro G, Crisafulli C. The biological pathways of Alzheimer disease: A review. AIMS Neuroscience. 2021;**3**(1):86-132

[16] Nikolac Perkovic M, Pivac N. Genetic markers of Alzheimer's disease. Advances in Experimental Medicine and Biology. 2019;**1192**:27-52

[17] Goldman JS, Hahn SE, Catania JW, LaRusse-Eckert S, Butson MB, Rumbaugh M, et al. Genetic counseling and testing for Alzheimer disease: joint practice guidelines of the American College of Medical Genetics and the National Society of Genetic Counselors. Genetics in Medicine : Official Journal of the American College of Medical Genetics. 2011;**13**(6):597-605

[18] Bekris LM, Yu CE, Bird TD, Tsuang DW. Genetics of Alzheimer disease. Journal of Geriatric Psychiatry and Neurology. 2010;**23**(4):213-227

[19] Skotte N. Genome-wide association studies identify new interesting loci for late-onset Alzheimer's disease. Clinical Genetics. 2010;**77**(4):330-332

[20] Chouraki V, Seshadri S. Genetics of Alzheimer's disease. Advances in Genetics. 2014;**87**:245-294

[21] Ghebremedhin E, Schultz C, Braak E, Braak H. High frequency of apolipoprotein E epsilon4 allele in young individuals with very mild Alzheimer's disease-related neurofibrillary changes. Experimental Neurology. 1998;**153**(1):152-155

[22] Shi Y, Yamada K, Liddelow SA, Smith ST, Zhao L, Luo W, et al. ApoE4 markedly exacerbates tau-mediated neurodegeneration in a mouse model of tauopathy. Nature. 2017;**549**(7673): 523-527

[23] Yamazaki Y, Zhao N, Caulfield TR, Liu CC, Bu G. Apolipoprotein E and Alzheimer disease: Pathobiology and targeting strategies. Nature Reviews Neurology. 2019;**15**(9):501-518

[24] Ulrich JD, Ulland TK, Mahan TE, Nystrom S, Nilsson KP, Song WM, et al. ApoE facilitates the microglial response to amyloid plaque pathology. The Journal of Experimental Medicine. 2018;**215**(4):1047-1058

[25] Mahley RW. Apolipoprotein E: cholesterol transport protein with expanding role in cell biology. Science. 1988;**240**(4852):622-630

[26] Puglielli L, Tanzi RE, Kovacs DM. Alzheimer's disease: The cholesterol connection. Nature Neuroscience. 2003;**6**(4):345-351

[27] Harold D, Abraham R, Hollingworth P, Sims R, Gerrish A, Hamshere ML, et al. Genome-wide association study identifies variants at CLU and PICALM associated with Alzheimer's disease. Nature Genetics. 2009;**41**(10):1088-1093

[28] Lambert JC, Heath S, Even G, Campion D, Sleegers K, Hiltunen M, et al. Genome-wide association study identifies variants at CLU and CR1 associated with Alzheimer's disease. Nature Genetics. 2009;**41**(10): 1094-1099

[29] Saunders AM, Strittmatter WJ, Schmechel D, George-Hyslop PH, Pericak-Vance MA, Joo SH, et al. Association of apolipoprotein E allele epsilon 4 with late-onset familial and sporadic Alzheimer's disease. Neurology. 1993;**43**(8):1467-1472

[30] Farrer LA, Cupples LA, Haines JL, Hyman B, Kukull WA, Mayeux R, et al.

Effects of age, sex, and ethnicity on the association between apolipoprotein E genotype and Alzheimer disease. A meta-analysis. APOE and Alzheimer disease meta analysis consortium. JAMA. 1997;**278**(16):1349-1356

[31] Chen Y, Zhang J, Zhang B, Gong CX. Targeting insulin signaling for the treatment of Alzheimer's disease. Current Topics in Medicinal Chemistry. 2016;**16**(5):485-492

[32] Mahley RW, Huang Y. Apolipoprotein e sets the stage: Response to injury triggers neuropathology. Neuron. 2012;**76**(5): 871-885

[33] Zhong N, Weisgraber KH. Understanding the association of apolipoprotein E4 with Alzheimer disease: Clues from its structure. The Journal of Biological Chemistry. 2009;**284**(10):6027-6031

[34] Zhao J, Lu W, Ren Y, Fu Y, Martens YA, Shue F, et al. Apolipoprotein E regulates lipid metabolism and α-synuclein pathology in human iPSC-derived cerebral organoids. Acta Neuropathologica. 2021;**142**(5):807-825

[35] Zhang DF, Xu M, Bi R, Yao YG. Genetic analyses of Alzheimer's disease in China: Achievements and perspectives. ACS Chemical Neuroscience. 2019;**10**(2):890-901

[36] Andrews SJ, Fulton-Howard B, Goate A. Interpretation of risk loci from genome-wide association studies of Alzheimer's disease. The Lancet Neurology. 2020;**19**(4):326-335

[37] Bertram L, McQueen MB, Mullin K, Blacker D, Tanzi RE. Systematic meta-analyses of Alzheimer disease genetic association studies: The AlzGene database. Nature Genetics. 2007;**39**(1): 17-23

[38] Heneka MT, Carson MJ, El Khoury J, Landreth GE, Brosseron F, Feinstein DL, et al. Neuroinflammation in Alzheimer's disease. The Lancet Neurology. 2015;**14**(4):388-405

[39] Chen Z, Zhong C. Oxidative stress in Alzheimer's disease. Neuroscience Bulletin. 2014;**30**(2):271-281

[40] Wang X, Wang W, Li L, Perry G, Lee HG, Zhu X. Oxidative stress and mitochondrial dysfunction in Alzheimer's disease. Biochimica et Biophysica Acta. 2014;**1842**(8): 1240-1247

[41] DuBoff B, Feany M, Gotz J. Why size matters - balancing mitochondrial dynamics in Alzheimer's disease. Trends in Neurosciences. 2013;**36**(6):325-335

[42] Godoy JA, Rios JA, Zolezzi JM, Braidy N, Inestrosa NC. Signaling pathway cross talk in Alzheimer's disease. Cell Communication and Signaling: CCS. 2014;**12**:23

[43] Dik MG, Jonker C, Comijs HC, Deeg DJ, Kok A, Yaffe K, et al. Contribution of metabolic syndrome components to cognition in older individuals. Diabetes Care. 2007; **30**(10):2655-2660

[44] Campos-Pena V, Toral-Rios D, Becerril-Perez F, Sanchez-Torres C, Delgado-Namorado Y, Torres-Ossorio E, et al. Metabolic syndrome as a risk factor for Alzheimer's disease: Is abeta a crucial factor in both pathologies? Antioxidants & Redox Signaling. 2017;**26**(10):542-560

[45] Whyte LS, Lau AA, Hemsley KM, Hopwood JJ, Sargeant TJ. Endo-lysosomal and autophagic dysfunction: A driving factor in Alzheimer's disease? Journal of Neurochemistry. 2017; **140**(5):703-717

[46] Pereira C, Agostinho P, Moreira PI, Cardoso SM, Oliveira CR. Alzheimer's disease-associated neurotoxic mechanisms and neuroprotective

strategies. Current Drug Targets CNS and Neurological Disorders. 2005;**4**(4): 383-403

[47] Gkanatsiou E, Nilsson J, Toomey CE, Vrillon A, Kvartsberg H, Portelius E, et al. Amyloid pathology and synaptic loss in pathological aging. Journal of Neurochemistry. 2021;**159**(2): 258-272

[48] Garcia-Osta A, Alberini CM. Amyloid beta mediates memory formation. Learning & Memory. 2009;**16**(4):267-272

[49] Palmeri A, Ricciarelli R, Gulisano W, Rivera D, Rebosio C, Calcagno E, et al. Amyloid-beta peptide is needed for cGMP-induced long-term potentiation and memory. The Journal of Neuroscience: The Official Journal of the Society for Neuroscience. 2017; **37**(29):6926-6937

[50] Hampel H, Hardy J, Blennow K, Chen C, Perry G, Kim SH, et al. The Amyloid-β Pathway in Alzheimer's Disease. Molecular Psychiatry. 2021 Aug 30. Epub ahead of print

[51] Zhang L, Guo XQ, Chu JF, Zhang X, Yan ZR, Li YZ. Potential hippocampal genes and pathways involved in Alzheimer's disease: A bioinformatic analysis. Genetics and Molecular Research: GMR. 2015;**14**(2):7218-7232

[52] Rauk A. Why is the amyloid beta peptide of Alzheimer's disease neurotoxic? Dalton Transactions. 2008;**10**:1273-1282

[53] Carrillo-Mora P, Luna R, Colin-Barenque L. Amyloid beta: multiple mechanisms of toxicity and only some protective effects? Oxidative Medicine and Cellular Longevity. 2014;**2014**:795375

[54] Sadigh-Eteghad S, Sabermarouf B, Majdi A, Talebi M, Farhoudi M, Mahmoudi J. Amyloid-beta: A crucial factor in Alzheimer's disease. Medical

Principles and Practice: International Journal of the Kuwait University, Health Science Centre. 2015;**24**(1):1-10

[55] Mukherjee P, Pasinetti GM. The role of complement anaphylatoxin C5a in neurodegeneration: implications in Alzheimer's disease. Journal of Neuroimmunology. 2000;**105**(2):124-130

[56] Luan K, Rosales JL, Lee KY. Viewpoint: Crosstalks between neurofibrillary tangles and amyloid plaque formation. Ageing Research Reviews. 2013;**12**(1):174-181

[57] Llanos-Gonzalez E, Henares-Chavarino AA, Pedrero-Prieto CM, Garcia-Carpintero S, Frontinan-Rubio J, Sancho-Bielsa FJ, et al. Interplay between mitochondrial oxidative disorders and proteostasis in Alzheimer's disease. Frontiers in Neuroscience. 2019;**13**:1444

[58] Butterfield DA, Bader Lange ML, Sultana R. Involvements of the lipid peroxidation product, HNE, in the pathogenesis and progression of Alzheimer's disease. Biochimica et Biophysica Acta. 2010;**1801**(8):924-929

[59] Cheignon C, Tomas M, Bonnefont-Rousselot D, Faller P, Hureau C, Collin F. Oxidative stress and the amyloid beta peptide in Alzheimer's disease. Redox Biology. 2018; **14**:450-464

[60] Chen YY, Yu XY, Chen L, Vaziri ND, Ma SC, Zhao YY. Redox signaling in aging kidney and opportunity for therapeutic intervention through natural products. Free Radical Biology & Medicine. 2019;**141**:141-149

[61] Bruce-Keller AJ, Gupta S, Knight AG, Beckett TL, McMullen JM, Davis PR, et al. Cognitive impairment in humanized APPxPS1 mice is linked to Abeta(1-42) and NOX activation. Neurobiology of Disease. 2011;**44**(3): 317-326

[62] Kothari V, Luo Y, Tornabene T, O'Neill AM, Greene MW, Geetha T, et al. High fat diet induces brain insulin resistance and cognitive impairment in mice. Biochimica et Biophysica Acta Molecular Basis of Disease. 2017; **1863**(2):499-508

[63] Wong KY, Roy J, Fung ML, Heng BC, Zhang C, Lim LW. Relationships between mitochondrial dysfunction and neurotransmission failure in Alzheimer's disease. Aging and Disease. 2020;**11**(5):1291-1316

[64] Swerdlow RH, Khan SM. A "mitochondrial cascade hypothesis" for sporadic Alzheimer's disease. Medical Hypotheses. 2004;**63**(1):8-20

[65] Liu Y, Liu F, Iqbal K, Grundke-Iqbal I, Gong CX. Decreased glucose transporters correlate to abnormal hyperphosphorylation of tau in Alzheimer disease. FEBS Letters. 2008;**582**(2):359-364

[66] Nikinmaa M, Pursiheimo S, Soitamo AJ. Redox state regulates HIF-1alpha and its DNA binding and phosphorylation in salmonid cells. Journal of Cell Science. 2004;**117** (Pt 15):3201-3206

[67] Morris G, Walder K, Puri BK, Berk M, Maes M. The deleterious effects of oxidative and nitrosative stress on palmitoylation, membrane lipid rafts and lipid-based cellular signalling: New drug targets in neuroimmune disorders. Molecular Neurobiology. 2016;**53**(7): 4638-4658

[68] Pena-Bautista C, Baquero M, Vento M, Chafer-Pericas C. Free radicals in Alzheimer's disease: Lipid peroxidation biomarkers. Clinica Chimica Acta. 2019;**491**:85-90

[69] Zou Y, Watters A, Cheng N, Perry CE, Xu K, Alicea GM, et al. Polyunsaturated fatty acids from astrocytes activate PPARgamma signaling in cancer cells to promote brain metastasis. Cancer Discovery. 2019;**9**(12):1720-1735

[70] Benseny-Cases N, Klementieva O, Cotte M, Ferrer I, Cladera J. Microspectroscopy (muFTIR) reveals co-localization of lipid oxidation and amyloid plaques in human Alzheimer disease brains. Analytical Chemistry. 2014;**86**(24):12047-12054

[71] Montine TJ, Neely MD, Quinn JF, Beal MF, Markesbery WR, Roberts LJ, et al. Lipid peroxidation in aging brain and Alzheimer's disease. Free Radical Biology & Medicine. 2002;**33**(5): 620-626

[72] Marnett LJ. Lipid peroxidation-DNA damage by malondialdehyde. Mutation Research. 1999;**424**(1-2): 83-95

[73] Kao YC, Ho PC, Tu YK, Jou IM, Tsai KJ. Lipids and Alzheimer's disease. International Journal of Molecular Sciences. 2020;**21**(4):1505

[74] Doyle R, Sadlier DM, Godson C. Pro-resolving lipid mediators: Agents of anti-ageing? Seminars in Immunology. 2018;**40**:36-48

[75] Chaney A, Williams SR, Boutin H. In vivo molecular imaging of neuroinflammation in Alzheimer's disease. Journal of Neurochemistry. 2019;**149**(4):438-451

[76] Zotova E, Nicoll JA, Kalaria R, Holmes C, Boche D. Inflammation in Alzheimer's disease: Relevance to pathogenesis and therapy. Alzheimer's Research & Therapy. 2010;**2**(1):1

[77] Cunningham C. Microglia and neurodegeneration: The role of systemic inflammation. Glia. 2013;**61**(1):71-90

[78] Wang JH, Cheng XR, Zhang XR, Wang TX, Xu WJ, Li F, et al. Neuroendocrine immunomodulation network dysfunction in SAMP8 mice and PrP-hAbetaPPswe/PS1DeltaE9

mice: Potential mechanism underlying cognitive impairment. Oncotarget. 2016;7(17):22988-23005

[79] Mandrekar-Colucci S, Landreth GE. Microglia and inflammation in Alzheimer's disease. CNS & Neurological Disorders Drug Targets. 2010;9(2):156-167

[80] Ferreira ST, Clarke JR, Bomfim TR, De Felice FG. Inflammation, defective insulin signaling, and neuronal dysfunction in Alzheimer's disease. Alzheimer's & Dementia: The Journal of the Alzheimer's Association. 2014; 10(1 Suppl):S76-S83

[81] Kinney JW, Bemiller SM, Murtishaw AS, Leisgang AM, Salazar AM, Lamb BT. Inflammation as a central mechanism in Alzheimer's disease. Alzheimer's & Dementia. 2018;4:575-590

[82] Rubio-Perez JM, Morillas-Ruiz JM. A review: Inflammatory process in Alzheimer's disease, role of cytokines. The Scientific World Journal. 2012;2012:756357

[83] Trojan E, Tylek K, Schroder N, Kahl I, Brandenburg LO, Mastromarino M, et al. The N-formyl peptide receptor 2 (FPR2) agonist MR-39 improves ex vivo and in vivo amyloid beta (1-42)-induced neuroinflammation in mouse models of Alzheimer's disease. Molecular Neurobiology. 2021;58(12): 6203-6221

[84] Kim DJ, Kim YS. Trimethyltin-induced microglial activation via NADPH oxidase and MAPKs pathway in BV-2 microglial cells. Mediators of Inflammation. 2015;2015:729509

[85] Sutinen EM, Pirttila T, Anderson G, Salminen A, Ojala JO. Pro-inflammatory interleukin-18 increases Alzheimer's disease-associated amyloid-beta production in human neuron-like cells.

Journal of Neuroinflammation. 2012; 9:199

[86] Sutinen EM, Korolainen MA, Hayrinen J, Alafuzoff I, Petratos S, Salminen A, et al. Interleukin-18 alters protein expressions of neurodegenerative diseases-linked proteins in human SH-SY5Y neuron-like cells. Frontiers in Cellular Neuroscience. 2014;8:214

[87] Oakley R, Tharakan B. Vascular hyperpermeability and aging. Aging and Disease. 2014;5(2):114-125

[88] Escartin C, Galea E, Lakatos A, O'Callaghan JP, Petzold GC, Serrano-Pozo A, et al. Reactive astrocyte nomenclature, definitions, and future directions. Nature Neuroscience. 2021;24(3):312-325

[89] Yamamoto M, Kiyota T, Horiba M, Buescher JL, Walsh SM, Gendelman HE, et al. Interferon-gamma and tumor necrosis factor-alpha regulate amyloid-beta plaque deposition and beta-secretase expression in Swedish mutant APP transgenic mice. The American Journal of Pathology. 2007;170(2): 680-692

[90] Ojala JO, Sutinen EM, Salminen A, Pirttila T. Interleukin-18 increases expression of kinases involved in tau phosphorylation in SH-SY5Y neuroblastoma cells. Journal of Neuroimmunology. 2008;205(1-2): 86-93

[91] Quintanilla RA, Orellana DI, Gonzalez-Billault C, Maccioni RB. Interleukin-6 induces Alzheimer-type phosphorylation of tau protein by deregulating the cdk5/p35 pathway. Experimental Cell Research. 2004; 295(1):245-257

[92] Chitnis T, Weiner HL. CNS inflammation and neurodegeneration. The Journal of Clinical Investigation. 2017;127(10):3577-3587

[93] Ahmed A, Patil AA, Agrawal DK. Immunobiology of spinal cord injuries and potential therapeutic approaches. Molecular and Cellular Biochemistry. 2018;**441**(1-2):181-189

[94] Hong S, Beja-Glasser VF, Nfonoyim BM, Frouin A, Li S, Ramakrishnan S, et al. Complement and microglia mediate early synapse loss in Alzheimer mouse models. Science. 2016;**352**(6286):712-716

[95] Stephan AH, Barres BA, Stevens B. The complement system: An unexpected role in synaptic pruning during development and disease. Annual Review of Neuroscience. 2012;**35**:369-389

[96] Munoz P, Ardiles AO, Perez-Espinosa B, Nunez-Espinosa C, Paula-Lima A, Gonzalez-Billault C, et al. Redox modifications in synaptic components as biomarkers of cognitive status, in brain aging and disease. Mechanisms of Ageing and Development. 2020;**189**:111250

[97] Del Prete D, Checler F, Chami M. Ryanodine receptors: Physiological function and deregulation in Alzheimer disease. Molecular Neurodegeneration. 2014;**9**:21

[98] Welser-Alves JV, Milner R. Microglia are the major source of TNF-alpha and TGF-beta1 in postnatal glial cultures; regulation by cytokines, lipopolysaccharide, and vitronectin. Neurochemistry International. 2013;**63**(1):47-53

[99] Gajardo I, Salazar CS, Lopez-Espindola D, Estay C, Flores-Munoz C, Elgueta C, et al. Lack of pannexin 1 alters synaptic GluN2 subunit composition and spatial reversal learning in mice. Frontiers in Molecular Neuroscience. 2018;**11**:114

[100] Flores-Munoz C, Gomez B, Mery E, Mujica P, Gajardo I, Cordova C,

et al. Acute pannexin 1 blockade mitigates early synaptic plasticity defects in a mouse model of Alzheimer's disease. Frontiers in Cellular Neuroscience. 2020;**14**:46

[101] Hidalgo C, Arias-Cavieres A. Calcium, reactive oxygen species, and synaptic plasticity. Physiology. 2016;**31**(3):201-215

[102] SanMartin CD, Veloso P, Adasme T, Lobos P, Bruna B, Galaz J, et al. RyR2-mediated Ca(2+) release and mitochondrial ROS generation partake in the synaptic dysfunction caused by amyloid beta peptide oligomers. Frontiers in Molecular Neuroscience. 2017;**10**:115

[103] Munoz Y, Paula-Lima AC, Nunez MT. Reactive oxygen species released from astrocytes treated with amyloid beta oligomers elicit neuronal calcium signals that decrease phospho-Ser727-STAT3 nuclear content. Free Radical Biology & Medicine. 2018;**117**:132-144

[104] Allen NJ, Eroglu C. Cell Biology of astrocyte-synapse interactions. Neuron. 2017;**96**(3):697-708

[105] Gottfries CG, Bartfai T, Carlsson A, Eckernas S, Svennerholm L. Multiple biochemical deficits in both gray and white matter of Alzheimer brains. Progress in Neuro-Psychopharmacology & Biological Psychiatry. 1986;**10**(3-5):405-413

[106] Storga D, Vrecko K, Birkmayer JG, Reibnegger G. Monoaminergic neurotransmitters, their precursors and metabolites in brains of Alzheimer patients. Neuroscience Letters. 1996;**203**(1):29-32

[107] Arai H, Ichimiya Y, Kosaka K, Moroji T, Iizuka R. Neurotransmitter changes in early- and late-onset Alzheimer-type dementia. Progress in Neuro-Psychopharmacology &

Biological Psychiatry. 1992;**16**(6): 883-890

[108] Lanari A, Amenta F, Silvestrelli G, Tomassoni D, Parnetti L. Neurotransmitter deficits in behavioural and psychological symptoms of Alzheimer's disease. Mechanisms of Ageing and Development. 2006; **127**(2):158-165

[109] Nobili A, Latagliata EC, Viscomi MT, Cavallucci V, Cutuli D, Giacovazzo G, et al. Dopamine neuronal loss contributes to memory and reward dysfunction in a model of Alzheimer's disease. Nature Communications. 2017;**8**:14727

[110] Chalermpalanupap T, Kinkead B, Hu WT, Kummer MP, Hammerschmidt T, Heneka MT, et al. Targeting norepinephrine in mild cognitive impairment and Alzheimer's disease. Alzheimer's Research & Therapy. 2013;**5**(2):21

[111] Parikh V, Bangasser DA. Cholinergic signaling dynamics and cognitive control of attention. Current Topics in Behavioral Neurosciences. 2020;**45**:71-87

[112] Woolf NJ, Butcher LL. Cholinergic systems mediate action from movement to higher consciousness. Behavioural Brain Research. 2011;**221**(2):488-498

[113] Cheng YJ, Lin CH, Lane HY. Involvement of cholinergic, adrenergic, and glutamatergic network modulation with cognitive dysfunction in Alzheimer's disease. International Journal of Molecular Sciences. 2021;**22**(5):2283

[114] Baker-Nigh A, Vahedi S, Davis EG, Weintraub S, Bigio EH, Klein WL, et al. Neuronal amyloid-beta accumulation within cholinergic basal forebrain in ageing and Alzheimer's disease. Brain: A Journal of Neurology. 2015;**138** (Pt 6):1722-1737

[115] Bracco L, Bessi V, Padiglioni S, Marini S, Pepeu G. Do cholinesterase inhibitors act primarily on attention deficit? A naturalistic study in Alzheimer's disease patients. Journal of Alzheimer's Disease: JAD. 2014; **40**(3):737-742

[116] Miao J, Shi R, Li L, Chen F, Zhou Y, Tung YC, et al. Pathological Tau from Alzheimer's brain induces site-specific hyperphosphorylation and SDS- and reducing agent-resistant aggregation of Tau in vivo. Frontiers in Aging Neuroscience. 2019;**11**:34

[117] Furcila D, DeFelipe J, Alonso-Nanclares L. A study of amyloid-beta and phosphotau in plaques and neurons in the hippocampus of Alzheimer's disease patients. Journal of Alzheimer's Disease: JAD. 2018;**64**(2):417-435

[118] Nie HZ, Shi S, Lukas RJ, Zhao WJ, Sun YN, Yin M. Activation of alpha7 nicotinic receptor affects APP processing by regulating secretase activity in SH-EP1-alpha7 nAChR-hAPP695 cells. Brain Research. 2010;**1356**:112-120

[119] Hefter D, Ludewig S, Draguhn A, Korte M. Amyloid, APP, and electrical activity of the brain. The Neuroscientist A Review Journal Bringing Neurobiology, Neurology and Psychiatry. 2020;**26**(3):231-251

[120] Picciotto MR, Caldarone BJ, King SL, Zachariou V. Nicotinic receptors in the brain. Links between molecular biology and behavior. Neuropsychopharmacology: Official Publication of the American College of Neuropsychopharmacology. 2000; **22**(5):451-465

[121] Tropea MR, Li Puma DD, Melone M, Gulisano W, Arancio O, Grassi C, et al. Genetic deletion of alpha7 nicotinic acetylcholine receptors induces an age-dependent Alzheimer's

disease-like pathology. Progress in Neurobiology. 2021;**206**:102154

[122] Zhao C, Zhang H, Li H, Lv C, Liu X, Li Z, et al. Geniposide ameliorates cognitive deficits by attenuating the cholinergic defect and amyloidosis in middle-aged Alzheimer model mice. Neuropharmacology. 2017;**116**:18-29

[123] Babaei P. NMDA and AMPA receptors dysregulation in Alzheimer's disease. European Journal of Pharmacology. 2021;**908**:174310

[124] Liu J, Chang L, Song Y, Li H, Wu Y. The role of NMDA receptors in Alzheimer's disease. Frontiers in Neuroscience. 2019;**13**:43

[125] Nygaard HB. Targeting fyn kinase in Alzheimer's disease. Biological Psychiatry. 2018;**83**(4):369-376

[126] Lopez-Bayghen E, Ortega A. Glial glutamate transporters: new actors in brain signaling. IUBMB Life. 2011;**63**(10):816-823

[127] Price BR, Johnson LA, Norris CM. Reactive astrocytes: The nexus of pathological and clinical hallmarks of Alzheimer's disease. Ageing Research Reviews. 2021;**68**:101335

[128] Carvajal FJ, Mattison HA, Cerpa W. Role of NMDA receptor-mediated glutamatergic signaling in chronic and acute neuropathologies. Neural Plasticity. 2016;**2016**:2701526

[129] Lu Y, Ren J, Cui S, Chen J, Huang Y, Tang C, et al. Cerebral glucose metabolism assessment in rat models of Alzheimer's disease: An 18F-FDG-PET study. American Journal of Alzheimer's Disease and Other Dementias. 2016;**31**(4):333-340

[130] Jeong DU, Oh JH, Lee JE, Lee J, Cho ZH, Chang JW, et al. Basal forebrain cholinergic deficits reduce glucose metabolism and function of cholinergic and GABAergic systems in the cingulate cortex. Yonsei Medical Journal. 2016;**57**(1):165-172

[131] Morrison BM, Lee Y, Rothstein JD. Oligodendroglia: metabolic supporters of axons. Trends in Cell Biology. 2013;**23**(12):644-651

[132] Garcia-Casares N, Jorge RE, Garcia-Arnes JA, Acion L, Berthier ML, Gonzalez-Alegre P, et al. Cognitive dysfunctions in middle-aged type 2 diabetic patients and neuroimaging correlations: a cross-sectional study. Journal of Alzheimer's Disease: JAD. 2014;**42**(4):1337-1346

[133] Rom S, Zuluaga-Ramirez V, Gajghate S, Seliga A, Winfield M, Heldt NA, et al. Hyperglycemia-driven neuroinflammation compromises BBB leading to memory loss in both diabetes mellitus (DM) type 1 and type 2 mouse models. Molecular Neurobiology. 2019;**56**(3):1883-1896

[134] Gaspar JM, Baptista FI, Macedo MP, Ambrosio AF. Inside the diabetic brain: Role of different players involved in cognitive decline. ACS Chemical Neuroscience. 2016;**7**(2):131-142

[135] Achari AE, Jain SK. Adiponectin, a therapeutic target for obesity, diabetes, and endothelial dysfunction. International Journal of Molecular Sciences. 2017;**18**(6):1321

[136] Akash MSH, Rehman K, Liaqat A. Tumor necrosis factor-alpha: Role in development of insulin resistance and pathogenesis of type 2 diabetes mellitus. Journal of Cellular Biochemistry. 2018;**119**(1):105-110

[137] Talbot K, Wang HY, Kazi H, Han LY, Bakshi KP, Stucky A, et al. Demonstrated brain insulin resistance in Alzheimer's disease patients is

associated with IGF-1 resistance, IRS-1 dysregulation, and cognitive decline. The Journal of Clinical Investigation. 2012;**122**(4):1316-1338

[138] Morales-Corraliza J, Wong H, Mazzella MJ, Che S, Lee SH, Petkova E, et al. Brain-wide insulin resistance, Tau phosphorylation changes, and hippocampal neprilysin and amyloid-beta alterations in a monkey model of type 1 diabetes. The Journal of Neuroscience: The Official Journal of the Society for Neuroscience. 2016; **36**(15):4248-4258

[139] Yamamoto N, Ishikuro R, Tanida M, Suzuki K, Ikeda-Matsuo Y, Sobue K. Insulin-signaling pathway regulates the degradation of amyloid beta-protein via astrocytes. Neuroscience. 2018;**385**:227-236

[140] Rojas-Carranza CA, Bustos-Cruz RH, Pino-Pinzon CJ, Ariza-Marquez YV, Gomez-Bello RM, Canadas-Garre M. Diabetes-related neurological implications and pharmacogenomics. Current Pharmaceutical Design. 2018;**24**(15): 1695-1710

[141] Pruzin JJ, Nelson PT, Abner EL, Arvanitakis Z. Review: Relationship of type 2 diabetes to human brain pathology. Neuropathology and Applied Neurobiology. 2018;**44**(4):347-362

[142] Yang Y, Wu Y, Zhang S, Song W. High glucose promotes Abeta production by inhibiting APP degradation. PLoS One. 2013;**8**(7): e69824

[143] Neth BJ, Craft S. Insulin resistance and Alzheimer's disease: Bioenergetic linkages. Frontiers in Aging Neuroscience. 2017;**9**:345

[144] Werther GA, Hogg A, Oldfield BJ, McKinley MJ, Figdor R, Allen AM, et al. Localization and characterization of insulin receptors in rat brain and pituitary gland using in vitro autoradiography and computerized densitometry. Endocrinology. 1987;**121**(4):1562-1570

[145] Ng RC, Chan KH. Potential neuroprotective effects of adiponectin in Alzheimer's disease. International Journal of Molecular Sciences. 2017;**18**(3):592

[146] Gabbouj S, Ryhanen S, Marttinen M, Wittrahm R, Takalo M, Kemppainen S, et al. Altered insulin signaling in Alzheimer's disease brain - special emphasis on PI3K-Akt pathway. Frontiers in Neuroscience. 2019;**13**:629

[147] Anderson NJ, King MR, Delbruck L, Jolivalt CG. Role of insulin signaling impairment, adiponectin and dyslipidemia in peripheral and central neuropathy in mice. Disease Models & Mechanisms. 2014;7(6):625-633

[148] Pena-Oyarzun D, Bravo-Sagua R, Diaz-Vega A, Aleman L, Chiong M, Garcia L, et al. Autophagy and oxidative stress in non-communicable diseases: A matter of the inflammatory state? Free Radical Biology & Medicine. 2018;**124**:61-78

[149] Alirezaei M, Kiosses WB, Flynn CT, Brady NR, Fox HS. Disruption of neuronal autophagy by infected microglia results in neurodegeneration. PLoS One. 2008;3(8):e2906

[150] Uddin MS, Stachowiak A, Mamun AA, Tzvetkov NT, Takeda S, Atanasov AG, et al. Autophagy and Alzheimer's disease: From molecular mechanisms to therapeutic implications. Frontiers in Aging Neuroscience. 2018;**10**:04

[151] He LQ, Lu JH, Yue ZY. Autophagy in ageing and ageing-associated diseases. Acta Pharmacologica Sinica. 2013;**34**(5):605-611

[152] Nilsson P, Saido TC. Dual roles for autophagy: Degradation and secretion of Alzheimer's disease abeta peptide. BioEssays. 2014;**36**(6):570-578

[153] Friedman LG, Qureshi YH, Yu WH. Promoting autophagic clearance: Viable therapeutic targets in Alzheimer's disease. Neurotherapeutics: The Journal of the American Society for Experimental NeuroTherapeutics. 2015;**12**(1):94-108

[154] Li Q, Liu Y, Sun M. Autophagy and Alzheimer's disease. Cellular and Molecular Neurobiology. 2017;**37**(3): 377-388

[155] Nixon RA, Wegiel J, Kumar A, Yu WH, Peterhoff C, Cataldo A, et al. Extensive involvement of autophagy in Alzheimer disease: An immuno-electron microscopy study. Journal of Neuropathology and Experimental Neurology. 2005;**64**(2):113-122

[156] Boland B, Kumar A, Lee S, Platt FM, Wegiel J, Yu WH, et al. Autophagy induction and autophagosome clearance in neurons: relationship to autophagic pathology in Alzheimer's disease. The Journal of Neuroscience: The Official Journal of the Society for Neuroscience. 2008;**28**(27):6926-6937

[157] Yu WH, Kumar A, Peterhoff C, Shapiro Kulnane L, Uchiyama Y, Lamb BT, et al. Autophagic vacuoles are enriched in amyloid precursor protein-secretase activities: Implications for beta-amyloid peptide over-production and localization in Alzheimer's disease. The International Journal of Biochemistry & Cell Biology. 2004; **36**(12):2531-2540

[158] Mizushima N. A(beta) generation in autophagic vacuoles. The Journal of Cell Biology. 2005;**171**(1):15-17

[159] SF F, Marcellino BK, Yue Z. Cell "self-eating" (autophagy) mechanism in Alzheimer's disease. The Mount Sinai Journal of Medicine, New York. 2010;**77**(1):59-68

[160] Silva DF, Esteves AR, Oliveira CR, Cardoso SM. Mitochondria: The common upstream driver of amyloid-beta and tau pathology in Alzheimer's disease. Current Alzheimer Research. 2011;**8**(5):563-572

[161] Silva MC, Nandi GA, Tentarelli S, Gurrell IK, Jamier T, Lucente D, et al. Prolonged tau clearance and stress vulnerability rescue by pharmacological activation of autophagy in tauopathy neurons. Nature Communications. 2020;**11**(1):3258

[162] Liu J, Li L. Targeting autophagy for the treatment of Alzheimer's disease: Challenges and opportunities. Frontiers in Molecular Neuroscience. 2019;**12**:203

[163] Scherz-Shouval R, Shvets E, Fass E, Shorer H, Gil L, Elazar Z. Reactive oxygen species are essential for autophagy and specifically regulate the activity of Atg4. The EMBO Journal. 2007;**26**(7):1749-1760

[164] Ji ZS, Mullendorff K, Cheng IH, Miranda RD, Huang Y, Mahley RW. Reactivity of apolipoprotein E4 and amyloid beta peptide: Lysosomal stability and neurodegeneration. The Journal of Biological Chemistry. 2006;**281**(5):2683-2692

[165] Inoue K, Rispoli J, Kaphzan H, Klann E, Chen EI, Kim J, et al. Macroautophagy deficiency mediates age-dependent neurodegeneration through a phospho-tau pathway. Molecular Neurodegeneration. 2012;**7**:48

[166] Nilsson P, Sekiguchi M, Akagi T, Izumi S, Komori T, Hui K, et al. Autophagy-related protein 7 deficiency in amyloid beta (Abeta) precursor protein transgenic mice decreases Abeta in the multivesicular bodies and induces

Abeta accumulation in the Golgi. The American Journal of Pathology. 2015;**185**(2):305-313

[167] Carvalho C, Santos MS, Oliveira CR, Moreira PI. Alzheimer's disease and type 2 diabetes-related alterations in brain mitochondria, autophagy and synaptic markers. Biochimica et Biophysica Acta. 2015;**1852**(8):1665-1675

[168] Pickford F, Masliah E, Britschgi M, Lucin K, Narasimhan R, Jaeger PA, et al. The autophagy-related protein beclin 1 shows reduced expression in early Alzheimer disease and regulates amyloid beta accumulation in mice. The Journal of Clinical Investigation. 2008;**118**(6):2190-2199

[169] Zhou X, Zhou J, Li X, Guo C, Fang T, Chen Z. GSK-3beta inhibitors suppressed neuroinflammation in rat cortex by activating autophagy in ischemic brain injury. Biochemical and Biophysical Research Communications. 2011;**411**(2):271-275

[170] Rohn TT, Vyas V, Hernandez-Estrada T, Nichol KE, Christie LA, Head E. Lack of pathology in a triple transgenic mouse model of Alzheimer's disease after overexpression of the anti-apoptotic protein Bcl-2. The Journal of Neuroscience: The Official Journal of the Society for Neuroscience. 2008;**28**(12):3051-3059

[171] Decuypere JP, Parys JB, Bultynck G. Regulation of the autophagic bcl-2/beclin 1 interaction. Cell. 2012;**1**(3):284-312

[172] Cai Z, Zhou Y, Liu Z, Ke Z, Zhao B. Autophagy dysfunction upregulates beta-amyloid peptides via enhancing the activity of gamma-secretase complex. Neuropsychiatric Disease and Treatment. 2015;**11**:2091-2099

[173] Qu J, Nakamura T, Cao G, Holland EA, McKercher SR, Lipton SA. S-Nitrosylation activates Cdk5 and contributes to synaptic spine loss induced by beta-amyloid peptide. Proceedings of the National Academy of Sciences of the United States of America. 2011;**108**(34):14330-14335

[174] Noble W, Olm V, Takata K, Casey E, Mary O, Meyerson J, et al. Cdk5 is a key factor in tau aggregation and tangle formation in vivo. Neuron. 2003;**38**(4):555-565

[175] Liu G, Wang H, Liu J, Li J, Li H, Ma G, et al. The CLU gene rs11136000 variant is significantly associated with Alzheimer's disease in Caucasian and Asian populations. Neuromolecular Medicine. 2014;**16**(1):52-60

[176] Shuai P, Liu Y, Lu W, Liu Q, Li T, Gong B. Genetic associations of CLU rs9331888 polymorphism with Alzheimer's disease: A meta-analysis. Neuroscience Letters. 2015;**591**:160-165

[177] Zhang P, Qin W, Wang D, Liu B, Zhang Y, Jiang T, et al. Impacts of PICALM and CLU variants associated with Alzheimer's disease on the functional connectivity of the hippocampus in healthy young adults. Brain Structure & Function. 2015;**220**(3):1463-1475

[178] Braskie MN, Jahanshad N, Stein JL, Barysheva M, McMahon KL, de Zubicaray GI, et al. Common Alzheimer's disease risk variant within the CLU gene affects white matter microstructure in young adults. The Journal of Neuroscience: The Official Journal of the Society for Neuroscience. 2011;**31**(18):6764-6770

[179] Beeg M, Stravalaci M, Romeo M, Carra AD, Cagnotto A, Rossi A, et al. Clusterin binds to Abeta1-42 oligomers with high affinity and interferes with peptide aggregation by inhibiting primary and secondary nucleation. The Journal of Biological Chemistry. 2016;**291**(13):6958-6966

[180] Mulder SD, Nielsen HM, Blankenstein MA, Eikelenboom P, Veerhuis R. Apolipoproteins E and J interfere with amyloid-beta uptake by primary human astrocytes and microglia in vitro. Glia. 2014;**62**(4): 493-503

[181] Letronne F, Laumet G, Ayral AM, Chapuis J, Demiautte F, Laga M, et al. ADAM30 downregulates APP-linked defects through cathepsin D activation in Alzheimer's disease. eBioMedicine. 2016;**9**:278-292

[182] Tian L, Zhang K, Tian ZY, Wang T, Shang DS, Li B, et al. Decreased expression of cathepsin D in monocytes is related to the defective degradation of amyloid-beta in Alzheimer's disease. Journal of Alzheimer's Disease: JAD. 2014;**42**(2):511-520

[183] Cheng S, Wani WY, Hottman DA, Jeong A, Cao D, LeBlanc KJ, et al. Haplodeficiency of cathepsin D does not affect cerebral amyloidosis and autophagy in APP/PS1 transgenic mice. Journal of Neurochemistry. 2017;**142**(2): 297-304

[184] Paz YMCA, Garcia-Cardenas JM, Lopez-Cortes A, Salazar C, Serrano M, Leone PE. Positive association of the cathepsin D Ala224Val gene polymorphism with the risk of Alzheimer's disease. The American Journal of the Medical Sciences. 2015;**350**(4):296-301

[185] Ntais C, Polycarpou A, Ioannidis JP. Meta-analysis of the association of the cathepsin D Ala224Val gene polymorphism with the risk of Alzheimer's disease: a HuGE gene-disease association review. American Journal of Epidemiology. 2004;**159**(6):527-536

[186] Ueda K, Fukushima H, Masliah E, Xia Y, Iwai A, Yoshimoto M, et al. Molecular cloning of cDNA encoding an unrecognized component of amyloid in Alzheimer disease. Proceedings of the National Academy of Sciences of the United States of America. 1993; **90**(23):11282-11286

[187] Majd S, Chegini F, Chataway T, Zhou XF, Gai W. Reciprocal induction between alpha-synuclein and beta-amyloid in adult rat neurons. Neurotoxicity Research. 2013;**23**(1): 69-78

[188] Roberts HL, Schneider BL, Brown DR. alpha-Synuclein increases beta-amyloid secretion by promoting beta−/gamma-secretase processing of APP. PLoS One. 2017;**12**(2):e0171925

[189] Giasson BI, Forman MS, Higuchi M, Golbe LI, Graves CL, Kotzbauer PT, et al. Initiation and synergistic fibrillization of tau and alpha-synuclein. Science. 2003; **300**(5619):636-640

[190] Oikawa T, Nonaka T, Terada M, Tamaoka A, Hisanaga S, Hasegawa M. alpha-synuclein fibrils exhibit gain of toxic function, promoting tau aggregation and inhibiting microtubule assembly. The Journal of Biological Chemistry. 2016;**291**(29):15046-15056

[191] Kerr JS, Adriaanse BA, Greig NH, Mattson MP, Cader MZ, Bohr VA, et al. Mitophagy and Alzheimer's disease: Cellular and molecular mechanisms. Trends in Neurosciences. 2017;**40**(3): 151-166

[192] Reddy PH, Oliver DM. Amyloid beta and phosphorylated tau-induced defective autophagy and mitophagy in Alzheimer's disease. Cell. 2019;**8**(5):488

[193] Hu Y, Li XC, Wang ZH, Luo Y, Zhang X, Liu XP, et al. Tau accumulation impairs mitophagy via increasing mitochondrial membrane potential and reducing mitochondrial Parkin. Oncotarget. 2016;**7**(14): 17356-17368

[194] Rothenberg C, Srinivasan D, Mah L, Kaushik S, Peterhoff CM, Ugolino J, et al. Ubiquilin functions in autophagy and is degraded by chaperone-mediated autophagy. Human Molecular Genetics. 2010;**19**(16): 3219-3232

[195] Zhang T, Jia Y. Meta-analysis of Ubiquilin1 gene polymorphism and Alzheimer's disease risk. Medical Science Monitor. 2014;**20**:2250-2255

[196] Yue Z, Wang S, Yan W, Zhu F. Association of UBQ-8i polymorphism with Alzheimer's disease in caucasians: A meta-analysis. The International Journal of Neuroscience. 2015;**125**(6): 395-401

[197] Natunen T, Takalo M, Kemppainen S, Leskelä S, Marttinen M, Kurkinen KMA, et al. Relationship between ubiquilin-1 and BACE1 in human Alzheimer's disease and APdE9 transgenic mouse brain and cell-based models. Neurobiology of Disease. 2016;**85**:187-205

[198] Stieren ES, El Ayadi A, Xiao Y, Siller E, Landsverk ML, Oberhauser AF, et al. Ubiquilin-1 is a molecular chaperone for the amyloid precursor protein. The Journal of Biological Chemistry. 2011;**286**(41):35689-35698

[199] Zhang M, Cai F, Zhang S, Zhang S, Song W. Overexpression of ubiquitin carboxyl-terminal hydrolase L1 (UCHL1) delays Alzheimer's progression in vivo. Scientific Reports. 2014;**4**:7298

[200] Guglielmotto M, Monteleone D, Boido M, Piras A, Giliberto L, Borghi R, et al. Abeta1-42-mediated down-regulation of Uch-L1 is dependent on NF-kappaB activation and impaired BACE1 lysosomal degradation. Aging Cell. 2012;**11**(5):834–844

[201] Puyal J, Ginet V, Grishchuk Y, Truttmann AC, Clarke PG. Neuronal autophagy as a mediator of life and death: Contrasting roles in chronic neurodegenerative and acute neural disorders. The Neuroscientist: A Review Journal Bringing Neurobiology, Neurology and Psychiatry. 2012; **18**(3):224-236

[202] Perluigi M, Di Domenico F, Butterfield DA. mTOR signaling in aging and neurodegeneration: At the crossroad between metabolism dysfunction and impairment of autophagy. Neurobiology of Disease. 2015;**84**:39-49

[203] Caccamo A, De Pinto V, Messina A, Branca C, Oddo S. Genetic reduction of mammalian target of rapamycin ameliorates Alzheimer's disease-like cognitive and pathological deficits by restoring hippocampal gene expression signature. The Journal of Neuroscience: The Official Journal of the Society for Neuroscience. 2014;**34**(23):7988-7998

[204] Caccamo A, Maldonado MA, Majumder S, Medina DX, Holbein W, Magri A, et al. Naturally secreted amyloid-beta increases mammalian target of rapamycin (mTOR) activity via a PRAS40-mediated mechanism. The Journal of Biological Chemistry. 2011;**286**(11):8924-8932

[205] She H, He Y, Zhao Y, Mao Z. Release the autophage brake on inflammation: The MAPK14/p38alpha-ULK1 pedal. Autophagy. 2018;**14**(6): 1097-1098

[206] Sole M, Esteban-Lopez M, Taltavull B, Fabregas C, Fado R, Casals N, et al. Blood-brain barrier dysfunction underlying Alzheimer's disease is induced by an SSAO/VAP-1-dependent cerebrovascular activation with enhanced Abeta deposition. Biochimica et Biophysica Acta Molecular Basis of Disease. 2019;**1865**(9): 2189-2202

[207] Sweeney MD, Sagare AP, Zlokovic BV. Cerebrospinal fluid

biomarkers of neurovascular dysfunction in mild dementia and Alzheimer's disease. Journal of Cerebral Blood Flow and Metabolism: Official Journal of the International Society of Cerebral Blood Flow and Metabolism. 2015;**35**(7):1055-1068

[208] de la Torre JC. Cardiovascular risk factors promote brain hypoperfusion leading to cognitive decline and dementia. Cardiovascular Psychiatry and Neurology. 2012;**2012**:367516

[209] Klohs J. An integrated view on vascular dysfunction in Alzheimer's disease. Neuro-Degenerative Diseases. 2019;**19**(3-4):109-127

[210] Popovic M, Laumonnier Y, Burysek L, Syrovets T, Simmet T. Thrombin-induced expression of endothelial CX3CL1 potentiates monocyte CCL2 production and transendothelial migration. Journal of Leukocyte Biology. 2008;**84**(1):215-223

[211] Carnevale D, Mascio G, D'Andrea I, Fardella V, Bell RD, Branchi I, et al. Hypertension induces brain beta-amyloid accumulation, cognitive impairment, and memory deterioration through activation of receptor for advanced glycation end products in brain vasculature. Hypertension. 2012;**60**(1):188-197

[212] Miller MC, Tavares R, Johanson CE, Hovanesian V, Donahue JE, Gonzalez L, et al. Hippocampal RAGE immunoreactivity in early and advanced Alzheimer's disease. Brain Research. 2008; **1230**:273-280

[213] Srikanth V, Maczurek A, Phan T, Steele M, Westcott B, Juskiw D, et al. Advanced glycation endproducts and their receptor RAGE in Alzheimer's disease. Neurobiology of Aging. 2011;**32**(5):763-777

[214] de la Torre J. The vascular hypothesis of Alzheimer's disease: A key to preclinical prediction of dementia using neuroimaging. Journal of Alzheimer's Disease: JAD. 2018; **63**(1):35-52

[215] Wierenga CE, Hays CC, Zlatar ZZ. Cerebral blood flow measured by arterial spin labeling MRI as a preclinical marker of Alzheimer's disease. Journal of Alzheimer's disease: JAD. 2014;**42**(Suppl 4):S411-S419

[216] Huang KL, Lin KJ, Ho MY, Chang YJ, Chang CH, Wey SP, et al. Amyloid deposition after cerebral hypoperfusion: Evidenced on [(18)F] AV-45 positron emission tomography. Journal of the Neurological Sciences. 2012;**319**(1-2):124-129

[217] Cho SJ, Yun SM, Jo C, Jeong J, Park MH, Han C, et al. Altered expression of Notch1 in Alzheimer's disease. PLoS One. 2019;**14**(11): e0224941

[218] Taylor KL, Henderson AM, Hughes CC. Notch activation during endothelial cell network formation in vitro targets the basic HLH transcription factor HESR-1 and downregulates VEGFR-2/KDR expression. Microvascular Research. 2002;**64**(3): 372-383

[219] Merlini M, Meyer EP, Ulmann-Schuler A, Nitsch RM. Vascular beta-amyloid and early astrocyte alterations impair cerebrovascular function and cerebral metabolism in transgenic arcAbeta mice. Acta Neuropathologica. 2011;**122**(3):293-311

[220] Duncombe J, Lennen RJ, Jansen MA, Marshall I, Wardlaw JM, Horsburgh K. Ageing causes prominent neurovascular dysfunction associated with loss of astrocytic contacts and gliosis. Neuropathology and Applied Neurobiology. 2017;**43**(6):477-491

[221] Sun MK, Alkon DL. The "memory kinases": Roles of PKC isoforms in signal

processing and memory formation. Progress in Molecular Biology and Translational Science. 2014;**122**:31-59

[222] Lucke-Wold BP, Turner RC, Logsdon AF, Simpkins JW, Alkon DL, Smith KE, et al. Common mechanisms of Alzheimer's disease and ischemic stroke: The role of protein kinase C in the progression of age-related neurodegeneration. Journal of Alzheimer's Disease: JAD. 2015;**43**(3): 711-724

[223] Alkon DL, Sun MK, Nelson TJ. PKC signaling deficits: A mechanistic hypothesis for the origins of Alzheimer's disease. Trends in Pharmacological Sciences. 2007;**28**(2):51-60

[224] de Barry J, Liegeois CM, Janoshazi A. Protein kinase C as a peripheral biomarker for Alzheimer's disease. Experimental Gerontology. 2010;**45**(1):64-69

[225] Wang H, Matsushita MT. Heavy metals and adult neurogenesis. Current opinion in Toxicology. 2021;**26**:14-21

[226] Inestrosa NC, Varela-Nallar L. Wnt signaling in the nervous system and in Alzheimer's disease. Journal of Molecular Cell Biology. 2014;**6**(1):64-74

[227] Wan W, Xia S, Kalionis B, Liu L, Li Y. The role of Wnt signaling in the development of Alzheimer's disease: A potential therapeutic target? BioMed Research International. 2014; **2014**:301575

[228] Popugaeva E, Pchitskaya E, Bezprozvanny I. Dysregulation of intracellular calcium signaling in Alzheimer's disease. Antioxidants & Redox Signaling. 2018;**29**(12):1176-1188

[229] Ruiz A, Matute C, Alberdi E. Endoplasmic reticulum Ca(2+) release through ryanodine and IP(3) receptors contributes to neuronal excitotoxicity. Cell Calcium. 2009;**46**(4):273-281

[230] Tong BC, Wu AJ, Li M, Cheung KH. Calcium Signaling in Alzheimer's Disease & Therapies. Biochimica et Biophysica Acta Molecular Cell Research. 2018;**1865**(11 Pt B): 1745-1760

[231] Berridge MJ. Inositol trisphosphate and calcium signalling mechanisms. Biochimica et Biophysica Acta. 2009;**1793**(6):933-940

[232] Jones PP, Braun AP. Store operated Ca2+ entry (SOCE): From structure to function. Channels. 2009;**3**(1):1-2

[233] Sushma MAC. Role of GPCR signaling and calcium dysregulation in Alzheimer's disease. Molecular and Cellular Neurosciences. 2019;**101**:103414

[234] Huang WJ, Zhang X, Chen WW. Role of oxidative stress in Alzheimer's disease. Biomedical Reports. 2016; **4**(5):519-522

[235] Hanger DP, Anderton BH, Noble W. Tau phosphorylation: The therapeutic challenge for neurodegenerative disease. Trends in Molecular Medicine. 2009;**15**(3):112-119

[236] Noble W, Hanger DP, Miller CC, Lovestone S. The importance of tau phosphorylation for neurodegenerative diseases. Frontiers in Neurology. 2013;**4**:83

[237] Wang JZ, Grundke-Iqbal I, Iqbal K. Kinases and phosphatases and tau sites involved in Alzheimer neurofibrillary degeneration. The European Journal of Neuroscience. 2007;**25**(1):59-68

[238] Liu F, Grundke-Iqbal I, Iqbal K, Gong CX. Contributions of protein phosphatases PP1, PP2A, PP2B and PP5 to the regulation of tau phosphorylation. The European Journal of Neuroscience. 2005;**22**(8):1942-1950

[239] Sontag E, Nunbhakdi-Craig V, Lee G, Brandt R, Kamibayashi C,

Kuret J, et al. Molecular interactions among protein phosphatase 2A, tau, and microtubules. Implications for the regulation of tau phosphorylation and the development of tauopathies. The Journal of Biological Chemistry. 1999;**274**(36):25490-25498

[240] Vogelsberg-Ragaglia V, Schuck T, Trojanowski JQ, Lee VM. PP2A mRNA expression is quantitatively decreased in Alzheimer's disease hippocampus. Experimental Neurology. 2001;**168**(2): 402-412

[241] Li L, Sengupta A, Haque N, Grundke-Iqbal I, Iqbal K. Memantine inhibits and reverses the Alzheimer type abnormal hyperphosphorylation of tau and associated neurodegeneration. FEBS Letters. 2004;**566**(1-3):261-269

[242] Martin L, Latypova X, Wilson CM, Magnaudeix A, Perrin ML, Terro F. Tau protein phosphatases in Alzheimer's disease: The leading role of PP2A. Ageing Research Reviews. 2013;**12**(1):39-49

[243] Mahaman YAR, Huang F, Embaye KS, Wang X, Zhu F. The Implication of STEP in synaptic plasticity and cognitive impairments in Alzheimer's disease and other neurological disorders. Frontiers in Cell and Development Biology. 2021;**9**:680118

[244] Lacor PN, Buniel MC, Chang L, Fernandez SJ, Gong Y, Viola KL, et al. Synaptic targeting by Alzheimer's-related amyloid beta oligomers. The Journal of Neuroscience: The Official Journal of the Society for Neuroscience. 2004;**24**(45):10191-10200

[245] Stevens TR, Krueger SR, Fitzsimonds RM, Picciotto MR. Neuroprotection by nicotine in mouse primary cortical cultures involves activation of calcineurin and L-type calcium channel inactivation. The Journal of Neuroscience: The Official

Journal of the Society for Neuroscience. 2003;**23**(31):10093-10099

[246] Kommaddi RP, Das D, Karunakaran S, Nanguneri S, Bapat D, Ray A, et al. Abeta mediates F-actin disassembly in dendritic spines leading to cognitive deficits in Alzheimer's disease. The Journal of Neuroscience: The Official Journal of the Society for Neuroscience. 2018;**38**(5):1085-1099

[247] Sala C, Piech V, Wilson NR, Passafaro M, Liu G, Sheng M. Regulation of dendritic spine morphology and synaptic function by Shank and Homer. Neuron. 2001; **31**(1):115-130

[248] Chen M, Huang N, Liu J, Huang J, Shi J, Jin F. AMPK: A bridge between diabetes mellitus and Alzheimer's disease. Behavioural Brain Research. 2021;**400**:113043

[249] Beurel E, Grieco SF, Jope RS. Glycogen synthase kinase-3 (GSK3): regulation, actions, and diseases. Pharmacology & Therapeutics. 2015;**148**:114-131

[250] Cai Z, Yan LJ, Li K, Quazi SH, Zhao B. Roles of AMP-activated protein kinase in Alzheimer's disease. Neuromolecular Medicine. 2012; **14**(1):1-14

[251] Bird TD. Genetic aspects of Alzheimer disease. Genetics in Medicine: Official Journal of the American College of Medical Genetics. 2008;**10**(4):231-239

[252] Li P, Marshall L, Oh G, Jakubowski JL, Groot D, He Y, et al. Epigenetic dysregulation of enhancers in neurons is associated with Alzheimer's disease pathology and cognitive symptoms. Nature Communications. 2019;**10**(1):2246

[253] Alcala-Vida R, Awada A, Boutillier AL, Merienne K. Epigenetic

mechanisms underlying enhancer modulation of neuronal identity, neuronal activity and neurodegeneration. Neurobiology of Disease. 2021;**147**:105155

[254] Amakiri N, Kubosumi A, Tran J, Reddy PH. Amyloid beta and MicroRNAs in Alzheimer's disease. Frontiers in Neuroscience. 2019;**13**:430

# Chapter 2

# An Innovative Framework for Integrative Rehabilitation in Dementia

*Valentin Bragin and Ilya Bragin*

## Abstract

Alzheimer's disease (AD) is a progressive neurodegenerative disorder with multiple pathophysiological mechanisms affecting every organ and system in the body. Cerebral hypoperfusion, hypoxia, mitochondrial failure, abnormal protein deposition, multiple neurotransmitters and synaptic failures, white matter lesions, and inflammation, along with sensory-motor system dysfunctions, hypodynamia, sarcopenia, muscle spasticity, muscle hypoxia, digestive problems, weight loss, and immune system alterations. Rehabilitation of AD patients is an emerging concept aimed at achieving optimum levels of physical and psychological functioning in the presence of aging, neurodegenerative processes, and progression of chronic medical illnesses. We hypothesize that the simultaneous implementation of multiple rehabilitation modalities can delay the progression of mild into moderate dementia. This chapter highlights recent research related to a novel treatment model aimed at modifying the natural course of AD and delaying cognitive decline for medically ill community-dwelling patients with dementia. For practical implementation of rehabilitation in AD, the standardized treatment protocols are warranted.

**Keywords:** dementia, Alzheimer's disease, vascular dementia, cerebrovascular disease, rehabilitation, physical exercises, nutrition, cognitive training, integrative treatment, pharmacological and non-pharmacological interventions

## 1. Introduction

Alzheimer's disease (AD) is a chronic and progressive neurodegenerative disorder, with multiple pathophysiological mechanisms. It currently affects more than 5 million individuals in the United States, and this number is growing daily. It is a whole-body disease, manifested by brain and body function changes during its progression. Clinically, people progressing through dementia demonstrate different manifestations of brain and body functions, including psychiatric manifestations, sensory-motor system disabilities, digestion insufficiency, and multiple bodily system involvement. A diverse combination of symptoms reflects the complexity of vascular, biochemical, physiological, and morphological changes in the brain and body during the development and progression of dementia. The amyloid cascade hypothesis has dominated the field of AD for many years. The intensive research concerning amelioration of the protein abnormalities in AD, based on the amyloid hypothesis, does not have practical value yet despite a very controversial, accelerated FDA approval of Aducanumab, an amyloid monoclonal antibody [1]. Conventional therapies—monotherapy or combinations of multiple medications—are not able to stop the progression of the disease and have very limited modifying effects. Our present understanding of the pathogenesis of AD goes far beyond brain dysfunction and pathology. Clinical and epidemiological studies have helped to identify modifiable factors in the onset and treatment of AD. Among these, hemodynamics, muscle health, and nutritional factors have been researched in animal and clinical studies for many years. The hemodynamic factor is related to vasculature, cerebral blood flow (CBF), and structural changes in the brain. A decrease in CBF is well documented during the progression of dementia. Sensory muscle status, changes in gait, balance, and fine dexterous motor skills are all strongly connected to the initiation and progression of dementia [2].

Nutritional deficiencies begin in the early stages of AD with a loss of taste and smell, which interferes with normal digestive processes. This disruption progresses to digestive disorders, malnutrition, and weight loss in advanced stages of dementia [3].

Rehabilitation is an important part of any treatment and has gained attention from the World Health Organization (WHO). In February 2017, there was a meeting hosted by the WHO, "Rehabilitation 2030: A Call for Action." At the event, WHO issued a call for action towards "concerted and coordinated global action to scale up rehabilitation." Rehabilitation is very important for people living on the wide spectrum of our world's economies and should thus be available for all medical conditions that require it, including dementia [4].

The rehabilitation of patients with dementia is an emerging concept aimed at achieving the optimum level of physical and psychological functioning in the progression of aging, neurodegenerative processes, and chronic medical illnesses. The general hypothesis for this combined therapy is based on the suggestion that every modality has a unique influence on brain functions in AD, and a combination of these modalities could have a synergistic effect, significantly slowing the rate of cognitive decline, improving quality of life, and delaying institutionalization. Nutrition and other non-pharmacological interventions, especially physical and cognitive activities, have shown promising results in delaying the onset of dementia and could potentially improve the outcome of dementia treatment. Research related to simultaneous implementation of medication and multiple non-pharmacological interventions is very limited [5, 6].

Studies relating to cognitive rehabilitation, physical exercises, and nutrition alone have shown a positive effect on cognition in animals and humans in time frames ranging from several months to several years [7–10].

Since 2000, we have developed a working rehabilitation model, utilizing all available resources, most of which are accessible to the average individual in the hopes of delaying the progression of dementia and possibly improving function in certain cognitive and physical domains. The objectives of this rehabilitation model are the activation of brain functions through the alteration of neurotransmitter activities and the increase of muscle activity, sensory input to the brain, CBF, and nutrients and oxygen supply.

To the best of our knowledge, there is no rehabilitation model related to the simultaneous implementation of multiple available modalities (medications, physical and cognitive exercises, nutrition, and sensory stimulations) for AD patients living at home. We hypothesize that the simultaneous implementation of all possible rehabilitation modalities could delay the progression of dementia significantly, when compared to the utilization of a single modality. Here, we present the key elements of this working rehabilitation model for patients living at home.

## 2. Pathophysiology of dementia in context of rehabilitation

### 2.1 Several factors in the pathogenesis of dementia

Our understanding of pathophysiology in dementia has shifted in focus from amyloid accumulation to hemodynamic and energetic metabolism changes in the brain. It is a chronic, progressive disorder that affects the entire body [11]. Amyloid accumulation in the brain is a dynamic process in response to different etiological factors: stress, hypoxia, loss of subcortical nuclei (the nucleus basalis of Meynert, the locus coeruleus, and the raphe nucleous) [12–14].

The hemodynamic factor is related to the development of hypoxia- and hypoxia-related metabolic and structural changes in the brain. Hypoperfusion affects white matter, subcortical nuclei, and the cortex of the brain in people with dementia. Chronic hypoxia decreases energy production in the brain, affecting protein synthesis pathways, which cause the development of reversible and irreversible morphological changes in the brain structure. During dementia progression, there are cerebral cortex and cortical corpus callosum atrophy, white matter damage, and dysfunction of subcortical nuclei. Alzheimer's dementia often begins as a disease of small blood vessels that are damaged by oxidation-induced inflammation and dysregulated amyloid metabolism, which may be seen as implications for early detection and therapy [15]. Today, there is an overlap between Alzheimer's disease and cerebral vascular dementia. Vast evidence from epidemiological, neural, physiological, clinical, and pharmacological studies suggests common pathogenic pathways between these two types of dementia and highlights the vital roles of vascular pathways in dementia development and pathology. The deficiency of cerebral blood flow could be a reason for neuronal dysfunction, white matter damage, and death of brain cells in both types of dementia.

The course of dementia is associated with progressive changes in cardiovascular pathology in the brain, increased numbers of micro and lacunar infarcts, cerebral atrophy, white matter changes, and signs of demyelination [16, 17]. CBF changes have been well documented in normal aging, MCI, and dementia by using different imaging techniques, such as single-photon emission computed tomography (SPECT), functional magnetic resonance imaging (fMRI), positron emission tomography (PET), among others. On an rCBF—SPECT test, people with mild AD showed a significant reduction in rCBF in the left parietal cortex during an episodic memory task [18]. The conversion from MCI to AD, as well as the progression of AD, is associated with CBF changes. The lower the patient's CBF, the faster and more drastic is their decline of Mini-Mental Status Exam (MMSE) scores [19].

The first notable changes in CBF start in the entorhinal and hippocampal areas of the brain, eventually expanding into the temporal and parietal lobes until finally reaching the frontal lobes [20]. In some places of the brain such as the sensory-motor strip areas and the cerebellum, CBF is relatively well-preserved in dementia [21]. This fact helps our understanding and explanation of the preservation of procedural memory in dementia, which is initiated in sensory-motor areas of the brain [22].

Moreover, judging from the same studies, it is quite possible to suggest that regulation of CBF is preserved as well, at least in the sensory-motor strip and cerebellum in moderate stages of the disease. Another example of preserved CBF in dementia is the report concerning increased CBF in frontal-occipital cortex in mild–moderate AD patients (7 affected people), compared to the control group (8 healthy individuals) during a visual face-matching task [23].

Energetic crises include mitochondrial failure and a decrease in the flow of substrate in brain neurons. A decrease in energy production in the central nervous

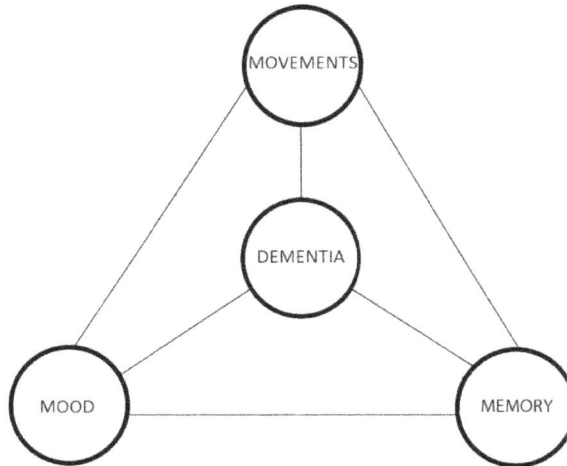

**Figure 1.**
*3M's dementia assessment model™ for dementia.*

system is one of the key factors in pathogenesis of dementia, which profoundly changes neuron function.

On the peripheral level, there are well-documented changes in sensory-motor system; decrease in feelings of taste, smell, and number of proprioceptive receptors; changes in mobility of joints and spine; increase in muscle spasticity; and decrease in muscles blood flow. Chronic muscles hypoxia is associated with muscle atrophy and sarcopenia. The decreased number of receptors and their functions result in diminished sensory input to the brain, and compromised CBF and neurotransmitters activities.

## 2.2 The 3M's dementia assessment model™ for dementia

Dementia has a progressive course of cognitive decline and physical disability, negatively affecting the quality of life, the capacity to socialize, and the ability to perform everyday activities. From a practical point of view, we developed the 3M's dementia assessment model™ for dementia evaluation, which includes assessing memory, mood, and movements. It is displayed in **Figure 1**.

Dementia can start from any of them, alone or in combination with each other. All factors could be affected at different speeds, and all of them have to be taken into consideration during dementia evaluation [24, 25]. Movements, general slowness, and fine motor skills could start before the development of the cognitive problems in dementia [26].

## 3. Modifiable factors in context of rehabilitation

Each of these modifiable factors could affect disease progression and treatment.

### 3.1 Stress

Acute and chronic stresses can affect brain and bodily functions by mobilization of sympathetic nervous system and activation of hypothalamic–pituitary–adrenal (HPA) axis on different stages of stress. Since Hans Selye's discovery of the general adaptation syndrome, countless publications demonstrate relationships between stressors, stress response, and diseases in animal and clinical studies [27]. Stress affects physiological and biochemical processes in every organ in the body during dementia initiation and progression [28]. Sensitivity to stress events increases with aging and may accelerate cognitive and physical decline in dementia [29]. Acute stress affects attention and memory [30]. Chronic stress could play a role in development and progression of dementia by persistent activation of fundamental surviving pathophysiological, mechanisms [31, 32]. There are links between chronic stress and level of memory loss in MCI and dementia [33]. Stress-related hormones mobilization is manifested in failures of homeostasis, thus leading to various diseases, including dementia [34]. Stress affects physiological and biochemical processes in every organ and system in the body during dementia initiation and progression [28].

They may be bidirectional relationships between stress and dementia. Stress is associated with CBF redistribution, mitochondrial and multiple neural pathways changes, and decreased attention and memory [35]. However, during dementia progression, loss of memory, behavior, and social communications could be stressors and evoke stress response by themselves.

There is related data utilization of different interventions aimed at modulation of stress response; the practical recommendations are in the early stages of research [36]. Effective stress management activities could be helpful for patients with dementia and their caregivers and need to be included in dementia treatment strategy [36, 37].

### 3.2 Depression and other emotional problems

Depression like dementia is a whole-body disease, affecting brain metabolism, sensory systems, muscle health, and nutrition. Depression could share common pathophysiological mechanisms with dementia, such as hypoperfusion, hypoxia, oxidative stress, and energetic and neurotransmitters failure and stress. Depression is one of the risk factors for developing dementia [24].

Depression could precede dementia and accompany dementia progression. The "vascular depression" hypothesis has been proposed, based on clinical, physiological, and morphological changes in seniors, suffering from persistent depression [38]. Clinical and radiology data and epidemiological studies demonstrate the changes in brain structure in dementia in old-old patients [39]. Treatment of late-life depression with vascular pathology is a challenging task for clinicians.

Apathy and anxiety may be seen in depression and dementia affecting the course of these diseases and associated with detrimental effects on activities of daily living [40–43].

### 3.3 CBF and vascular pathology

The fact that cardiovascular pathology occurs in multiple neurodegenerative processes in dementia is well documented. However, it remains necessary to investigate the interconnections and order of occurrence of these two factors [44, 45]. The course of dementia is associated with progressive changes in cardiovascular pathology, increased numbers of microbleeds and lacunar infarcts, cerebral atrophy, white matter changes, and signs of demyelination [17].

Vascular pathology and decrease of CBF contribute to progression of clinical manifestations, improving cognitive and physical functions, and developing morphological changes in dementia. Changes in CBF, cerebral ischemia, and hypoxia negatively affect substrate delivery, necessary for energy production and protein synthesis and essential neuronal activities [46].

### 3.4 Digestive system

In epidemiological studies, nutrition has been under investigation for many years as an important factor contributing to healthy aging and prevention of dementia and multiple chronic diseases.

For the purposes of this discussion, the nutritional aspect in the treatment of dementia can be separated into four components.

The first component is related to the diet. There is currently no consensus regarding a diet geared towards at least partially normalizing brain metabolism in dementia. Along with the well-known Mediterranean diet, calorie-restrictive diets, as well as ketogenic diets, may have a beneficial neuroprotective effect in aging and multiple neurodegenerative diseases [47]. The diet close to that used for cardiovascular pathology and diabetes with some modification geared towards very low carbohydrate products is probably the most suitable diet to be offered for dementia patients.

The second component is a number of vitamins and nutriceuticals, which have been known to affect critical biochemical pathways involved in the pathophysiology of dementia. Among them are vitamins and nutrients that are a part of the normal metabolic processes and become deficient during stress, lack of exercises, hypoxia, and many other clinical conditions. In a controlled study on institutionalized, moderate-to-severe dementia patients taking a vitamin/nutriceutical combination for 9 months demonstrated a significant delay in decline on the Dementia Rating Scale and clock-drawing test, compared to those receiving placebo. The vitamin-nutriceutical combination in this study was designed to support antioxidant activities, energy production, and protein synthesis. This small study supports the notion that even in severe dementia, there is still room for stabilization of disease progression [48]. The specific research data related to different nutritional substances and vitamins is out of scope of this chapter.

General recommendations include products that are rich in antioxidants and include dietary precursors for mitochondria function, protein metabolism, and membrane phosphatide synthesis [6, 49].

The third component is associated with changes in gastrointestinal functions in every part of the GI system. These begin in the early stages of dementia and worsen with disease progression, frequently manifested as nutritional disorders such as anorexia, poor digestion, malnutrition, and weight loss. The loss of taste and smell develops in the early stages of dementia, results in the loss of appetite, and negatively impacts all stages of digestion. Even in the early stages of AD, community-dwelling patients display poor nutritional consumption [50]. Patients with dementia often forget to eat or drink on time. In the advanced stages of dementia, progressive GI malfunctions occur simultaneously with chewing and swallowing problems, dysphagia, and a decreased feeling of thirst, all of which are connected to poor food digestion and absorption, vitamin deficiencies, decreased immunity, loss of muscle mass, increased frequency of infection, poor balance, and falls [3]. Weight loss is associated with severity and mortality in AD and is an indicator of protein, energy, vitamin, and nutrient deficiency [51]. According to these authors, in the middle stage of AD (MMSE—16.6 ± 4.9), significant weight loss is observed in more than 40% of patients living at home.

The presence of malnutrition in dementia could be a result of GI system dysregulation: changes in appetite, weight, and GI motility, and the probable development of exocrine pancreatic insufficiency.

An indicator of pancreatic exocrine insufficiency is the level of fecal elastase-1 in stool, the concentration of which decreases progressively with age. Pancreatic exocrine insufficiency was seen in 21.7% of people over 65 years without gastrointestinal disorders, surgery, or diabetes [52]. Pancreatic exocrine insufficiency is more prominent in patients with insulin-dependent diabetes [53].

The existence of pancreatic insufficiency during the aging process and in diabetes, as well as changes in glucose metabolism in dementia, makes it quite possible that exocrine pancreatic insufficiency plays an important role in the digestive malfunctions in dementia.

The fourth component is the microbiome. Imbalance in gut flora can negatively affect general health. The first connection between intestinal microbiome and longevity was described over a century ago by Elie Metchnikoff [54]. Research about the gut-brain axis demonstrates the strong bidirectional connections between gut–body health. Gut flora participates in production of serotonin, dopamine, and GABA—neurotransmitters, actively affected in many neurodegenerative illnesses and medical diseases as well. Stress, depression, and dementia negatively influence the health of the gut. A practical recommendation about using probiotics, prebiotics, and postbiotics for depression and dementia is on the horizon [55–57].

### 3.5 Medical illnesses

Medical illnesses (cardiac problems, diabetes, etc.) are risk factors for dementia development and progression. In recent years, accumulating evidence of research has suggested that cardiovascular pathology, especially irregular pulse, could be associated with dementia progression. In diabetes mellitus (type 2), there are metabolic changes, which affect vasculature and cell functions in every organ in the body. The cognitive and physical decline in dementia became worse with progression of diabetes.

The treatment and stabilization of these medical illnesses and disorders have a positive effect on people with dementia. The same approach could be applied to diseases related to the transport of oxygen to the organs (anemia, pulmonary pathology, and renal problems).

### 3.6 Cognitive activities

Mental activities have a positive effect on CBF in healthy individuals and have been shown to delay the onset of dementia [58]. Research related to improving CBF in AD patients through the use of cognitive activities is slowly growing. Recently a program of mental exercises for nursing home residents with mild AD showed an improvement in cognitive function after being implemented for 6 months. This program was based on extensive previous research done by the same research team relating to increased CBF during various mental tasks [59].

### 3.7 Physical activities

The connections between physical activities and rCBF are well established and done on healthy seniors, patients with MCI, and animal dementia models [60]. Physical exercise is considered a preventative or disease-modifying intervention, as it has shown a neuroprotective effect in brain aging [61]. Physical activities increase level of BDNF, which is responsible for brain health [62].

The effects of resistance training and aerobic exercises are connected to increased activity of the entire cardiovascular system and CBF simultaneously. These physical activities increase level of BDNF, which actively participate in learning, memory, and mood [63].

Hand exercises are more suitable and safer for fragile medically ill patients with all stages of AD because they can be done in a seated or laying position and appear to be a practical model for a home-based exercise regimen [11].

Simple hand movements have been shown to increase CBF in contralateral hemisphere of healthy subjects [64]. An increase in CBF during meditation, with simultaneous chanting and finger movements (dual tasks), has been observed by SPECT in healthy volunteers [65].

Physical activities have positive effect on neuropsychiatric symptoms in dementia [37].

Physical and mental exercises alone, as well as a combination of the both, could modify CBF and improve cerebral metabolism, decrease hypoxia, increase availability of oxygen and nutrients to brain cells and structures, increase brain vitality and prolong an active life for patients with dementia.

## 4. Rehabilitation model for dementia

Rehabilitation of AD patients is an emerging concept aimed at achieving optimum levels of physical cognitive and psychological functioning in the presence of neurodegenerative processes, aging, and progression of chronic medical illnesses.

Given the complexity regarding the pathogenesis of AD, we hypothesize that the simultaneous implementation of multiple rehabilitation modalities could delay the progression of dementia. To the best of our knowledge, there is no rehabilitation model designed for the treatment at home for many years. This program starts in the doctor's office and continues in the home indefinitely.

### 4.1 4M's dementia rehabilitation model™ for dementia

From a practical point of view, we approach dementia rehabilitation with the 4M's dementia rehabilitation model™, which includes treating memory, mood, movements, and mitochondria to increase the vitality of neurons and their connections by increasing CBF, as shown in **Figure 2**.

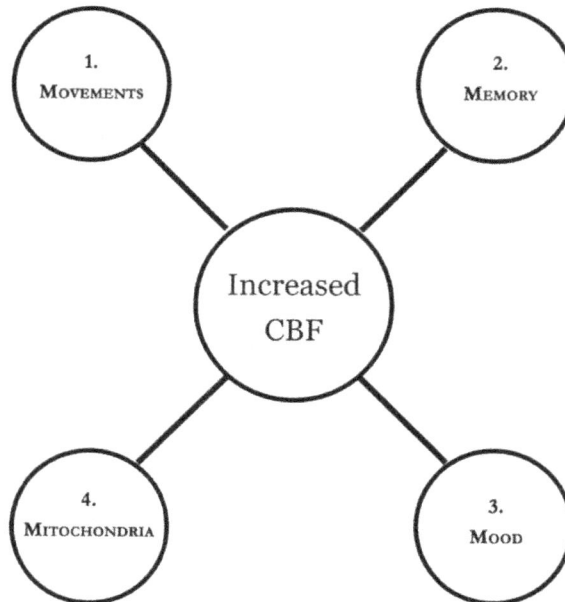

**Figure 2.**
*4M's dementia rehabilitation model™.*

## 4.2 Office and home parts of the program

The in-office part of the model includes (a) an assessment of cognitive functions and movements, with special attention paid to preserved areas in cognition and motor system; (b) education about AD, modifiable factors, which needs to be used; (c) teaching patients and caregivers stress reduction techniques, as well as appropriate physical and cognitive exercises, based on patient's level of dementia; (d) physical and cognitive training during office visits; and (e) monitoring of treatment progress during subsequent office visits.

The home part of the model includes (a) physical exercises, cognitive training, and stress management techniques practiced as per the workbook and videos (which are given to each patient); (b) sensory activation (light, sound, relaxation videos with tranquil nature scenery; and (c) nutrition.

The physical and cognitive aspects of the rehabilitation program have been developed based on the physiological, real-life interplay between physical activity, attention, and procedural memory. Physical activities require attention and help with procedural memory. All of them have a direct effect on CBF [64–66]. During the progression of AD, all three components deteriorate at different rates over time. However, they are relatively preserved, compared to other cognitive functions until the late stages of AD.

Over the years, preservation of cognitive function has been demonstrated up to 72 months of treatment. Remaining at the same level of cognitive function at the initial visit is a significant treatment achievement [67, 68].

Even though the progression of dementia is going along with development of chronic hypoxia, there is still room for developing neuroplastic changes in response to sensory-motor stimulation [69]. In recent review, ischemic damages evoke an initiation of network reorganization in spared areas of the brain [70].

## 4.3 Rehabilitation in chronic versus acute brain diseases

There are different goals for rehabilitation for chronic and acute brain diseases; even all available rehabilitation modalities are implemented simultaneously in both types of rehabilitation. The goal of rehabilitation in dementia is to prevent cognitive and physical decline and to preserve the level of functioning and the quality of life for as long as possible. Rehabilitation activities for people living at home have to continue without time limits, for many years. Home program refers to activities designed for joint patient and caregivers, which increase patient–caregiver connections. The office staff get training, related to interaction with patients and their caregivers. Much attention is placed on education and support of caregivers as well. Elements of physical, occupational, and speech therapy in outpatient clinics could be provided by office staff in the office and by caregivers at home. Cognitive and physical stabilization is expected, as demonstrated in **Figure 3**.

In stroke and head trauma (acute brain catastrophes), the goal of rehabilitation is to return to the premorbid level as close as possible. Rehabilitation in this case is

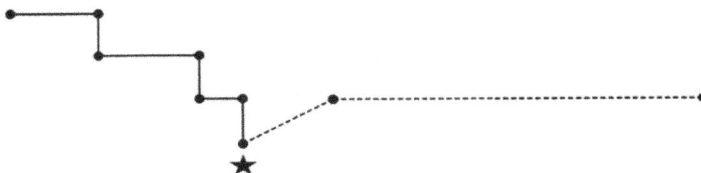

**Figure 3.**
*Rehabilitation in chronic brain disease.*

**Figure 4.**
*Rehabilitation in acute brain trauma/stroke.*

a time-limited process, lasting from several months to several years. Cognitive and physical improvement is expected, as shown in **Figure 4**.

**4.4 Six pillars of rehabilitation**

The six pillars of the program consist of pharmacological interventions, mild physical exercises, multisensory stimulation, cognitive training, nutrition, and emotional support. Each pillar has direct and indirect effects on the elements of the 4M's Dementia Rehabilitation Model™.

Medications and supplements comprise the first pillar in this model. Cholinesterase inhibitors, NMDA receptor antagonists, antidepressants, neuroleptics, and mood stabilizers, along with medication for sleep and pain, are used when clinically appropriate. Supplements include vitamin D3, B-complex, fish oil, folic acid, alpha-lipolic acid, acetyl-l-carnitine, inositol, Ribose, and other vitamins.

Mild physical exercises are the second pillar in this rehabilitation. Muscle activities couple with increasing brain blood flow and simultaneously attention and procedural memory training. Exercises are designed for people with extremely limited physical capacities and problems with gait and ambulation. The physical exercises are safe and done in sitting positions and can be performed in the doctor's office or at home.

Physical exercises mainly consist of simple, coordinated hand and leg exercises performed both with and without the use of simple objects, such as a tennis ball. Dual-task exercises consist of hand movements, coupled with counting and breathing. Special exercises have been developed for balance training and include eye movements for decreasing visual fields and working with neck movements.

Multisensory stimulations include pleasurable activities related to auditory, visual, and tactile and other sensory channels. For example, patients work on pegboards to increase finger mobility and right–left coordination, or patients read tongue twisters loudly, sing songs, or watch comedians.

Attention and memory training consist of computerized attention ("go, no-go") and working memory exercises ("N-back" paradigm), tasks that are performed in the doctor's office with different objects (words, numbers, shapes, pictures, textures) plus pen and paper cognitive exercises, performed at home.

Nutrition includes diet and digestive support for microbiome and pancreatic enzymes, if clinically indicated (loss of weight).

Emotional support consists of implementation of stress management tools, brief educational sessions, related to family relationships, psychotherapy for patient's emotional reactions in response to decline of cognitive and physical functions. For caregivers, there are psychotherapy sessions for developing coping strategies to manage behavior problems in dementia and to recognize symptoms of burnout syndrome. The family understanding and support help dementia victims stay at home for a long period of time.

## 5. Clinical cases

Here, we present two cases with mild dementia stabilized over years with an integrative treatment approach.

### 5.1 Case 1

Patient was an 87-year-old, retired engineer, who first came to our office at age 68. Her diagnosis was mild dementia with episodes of depression, anxiety, insomnia, HTN, diabetes, neuropathy, arthritis, dizziness, and gait problems. Her current psychiatric medications are memantine, gabapentin, clonazepam, zolpidem, buproprion SR, donepezil, vitamin D, lovaza, magnesium oxide, B-complex, and folic acid.

This patient has been treated for 19 years (2001–2020). Cognitive assessments include the MMSE, clock-drawing task, verbal fluency animals, and verbal fluency letters tests. She was doing full rehabilitation protocol with any new modifications, which had been developed during this time interval in our office.

As you can see in **Figures 5–8**, this patient has been stable for the whole period of treatment based on the results of these 4 tests.

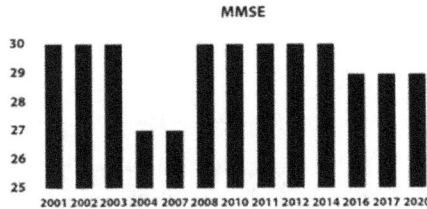

**Figure 5.**
*MMSE stabilization.*

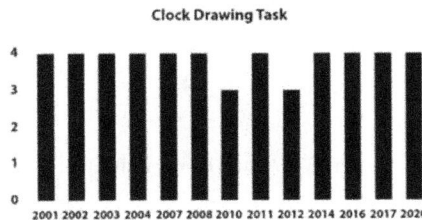

**Figure 6.**
*Clock-drawing task stabilization.*

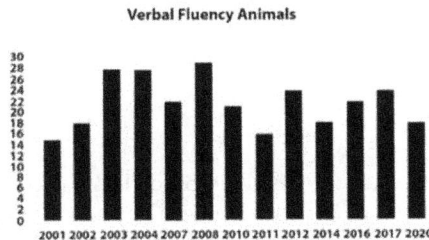

**Figure 7.**
*Verbal fluency animals.*

**Verbal Fluency Letters**

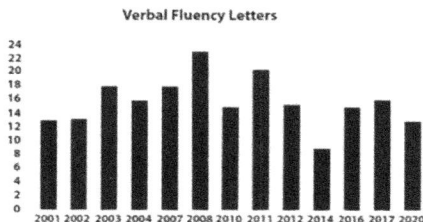

**Figure 8.**
*Verbal fluency letters.*

**MMSE**

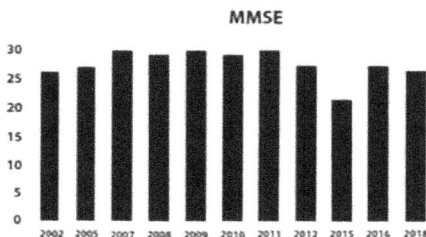

**Figure 9**
**MMSE stabilization.**

**Clock Drawing Task**

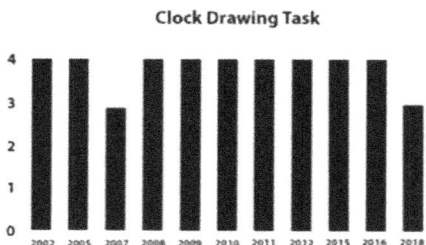

**Figure 10.**
*Clock-drawing task stabilization.*

**Verbal Fluency Animals**

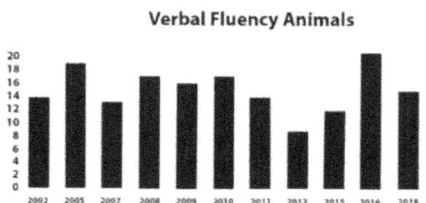

**Figure 11.**
*Verbal fluency animals.*

## 5.2 Case 2

This patient was a 92-year-old female, retired clerk, who came for treatment at age 74. Her diagnosis was mild dementia with episodes of depression, anxiety, insomnia, HTN, CAD, diabetes, arthritis, dizziness, and gait problems. She had a mini-stroke in 2015. Current medications are Namenda, Trintellix, B-complex, folic acid, and magnesium oxide.

**Verbal Fluency Letters**

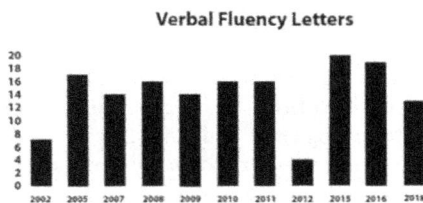

**Figure 12.**
*Verbal fluency letters.*

This patient has been treated for 16 years (2002–2020). Cognitive assessments include Mini-Mental Status Examination (MMSE), clock-drawing task, verbal fluency animals, and verbal fluency letters tests. She was doing full rehabilitation protocol with any new modifications as in the previous case 1.

After mini-stroke (2014–2015), her MMSE dropped to 22 and then returned to 25.

As you see in **Figures 9–12**, this patient has been stable for the whole period of treatment.


## 6. Discussion

The theoretical basis of this rehabilitation model is rooted in emerging research related to neuroplasticity data. Other well-known facts regarding AD pathogenesis—including chronic hypoperfusion and hypoxia, oxidative stress, and mitochondrial and bioenergetics failure—also provide a solid theoretical foundation upon which to effectively design and test different treatment modalities available for rehabilitation in AD [69–71]. Additionally, modifiable risk factors for AD development and progression continue to be identified [72].

In a broader sense, rehabilitation in AD could include medications that are available today (and those that will become available in the future), in addition to all possible non-pharmacological modalities that are aimed at stabilizing brain and body functions, with special attention to physical and cognitive exercises, sensory stimulations, and dietary modifications.

The rehabilitation of AD has to be seen as an ongoing treatment approach not limited by time constraints. It can be adapted to the different stages of this illness, including even the preclinical stage.

Not all motor and cognitive functions are equally affected in AD. At various levels of dementia and in each cognitive domain, there is a time-related evolution of brain disability. Meanwhile, there is a growing body of data related to the preservation of some of the brain functions in AD, including certain learning and procedural memory capacities, emotional and movement controls, and the ability to use external memory aids [72–76].

The multifaceted rehabilitation model for home usage presented here demonstrates strategies that go beyond the prescribing of medications to alleviate AD progression alone. It is a dynamic framework that is open to the addition of any newfound medications or innovations in nonpharmacological interventions. This model is based on a proactive, 24/7 approach to battling AD—starting with doctor's office visits and continuing into the patient's home for an indefinite period of time.

These rehabilitation strategies become meaningful only with ongoing support from caregivers who help the patients at home with nutrition and everyday physical and cognitive activities. This model is flexible, and the key to it is to use all the five elements of the program simultaneously. This kind of simultaneous approach is already commonly used in the treatment of many other progressive chronic ailments, such as cardiac problems, dyslipidemia, hypertension, and diabetes.

The cost for implementation of this home-based rehabilitation model is minimal (workbook, videos, and tennis ball). In addition, this model may ease the financial burden of this deadly disease on the health care system as a whole by reducing secondary medical problems from progressive dementia and delaying nursing home placement.

## 7. Conclusion

A multifaceted rehabilitation model for dementia at home offers a promising strategy for postponing cognitive and physical decline in dementia. Modifiable factors in dementia could be implemented at low cost.

The development of comprehensive therapy models for rehabilitation in dementia is a matter of time. There is an urgent need for the designing of long-term studies, in which all available modalities will be simultaneously implemented and for as long as possible. Further research is needed to assess the efficacy and economic impact of this multifaceted rehabilitation model.

## 8. Summary points

- Epidemiological studies have identified a number of modifiable factors in the onset and progression of dementia.

- A new understanding of the pathogenesis of dementia has revealed that protein changes in the brain develop simultaneously with cerebrovascular pathology.

- Progression of clinical dementia depends on the stress, emotional reactions, CBF, digestive system, medical illnesses profile, cognitive activities, and muscle health.

- Physical and mental activities may contribute to the delay of the onset of dementia and slow down the disease progression.

- A novel treatment model for dementia patients is the simultaneous use of nonpharmacological modifiable factors and pharmacological interventions for many years.

## Acknowledgements

Thank you to Vian Shekhtman and Nora Zagranichny for their assistance in preparation of this chapter.

## Conflict of interest

The authors declare that they have no competing interests. The authors have no financial interests in this project.

## Disclaimer

No grant support was received for this project.

## Notes/thanks

I want to thank the patients that have been treated in our center. Their participation and feedbacks were very valuable, and we are grateful for it.

Author details

Valentin Bragin[1*] and Ilya Bragin[1,2,3]

1 Stress Relief and Memory Training Center, New York, United States of America

2 St. Lukes University Health Network, Pennsylvania, United States of America

3 Lewis Katz School of Medicine at Temple University, Pennsylvania,
United States of America

*Address all correspondence to: val11235@gmail.com

IntechOpen

## References

[1] Golde TE. Disease modifying therapy for AD? Journal of Neurochemistry. 2006;**99**(3):689-707. DOI: 10.1111/j.1471-4159.2006.04211.x

[2] Sui SX, Williams LJ, Holloway-Kew KL, Hyde NK, Pasco JA. Skeletal muscle health and cognitive function: A narrative review. International Journal of Molecular Sciences. 2020;**22**(1):255. DOI: 10.3390/ijms22010255

[3] Pivi GA, Bertolucci PH, Schultz RR. Nutrition in severe dementia. Current Gerontology Geriatrics Research. 2012;**2012**:983056. DOI: 10.1155/2012/983056

[4] WHO Meeting Report. Rehabilitation 2030: A Call For Action. 2017. Available from: https://www.who.int/disabilities/care/Rehab2030MeetingRepor t_plain_text_version.pdf

[5] Ruthirakuhan M, Luedke AC, Tam A, Goel A, Kurji A, Garcia A. Use of physical and intellectual activities and socialization in the management of cognitive decline of aging and in dementia: a review. Journal of Aging Research. 2012;**2012**:384875. DOI: 10.1155/2012/384875

[6] Pocernich CB, Lange ML, Sultana R, Butterfield DA. Nutritional approaches to modulate oxidative stress in Alzheimer's disease. Current Alzheimer Research. 2011;**8**(5):452-469. DOI: 10.2174/156720511796391908

[7] Cicconetti P, Fionda A, Zannino G, Ettorre E, Marigliano V. Rehabilitation in Alzheimer's dementia. Recenti Progressi in Medicina. 2000;**91**:450-454

[8] Cotelli M, Calabria M, Zanetti O. Cognitive rehabilitation in Alzheimer's Disease. Aging Clinical and Experimental Research. 2006;**18**:141-143. DOI: 10.1007/BF03327429

[9] Manzine PR, Pavarini SCI. Cognitive rehabilitation: Literature review based on levels of evidence. Dementia Neuropsychology. 2009;**3**:248-255. DOI: 10.1590/S1980-57642009DN30300012

[10] Viola LF, Nunes PV, Yassuda MS, Aprahamian I, Santos FS, Santos GD, et al. Effects of a multidisciplinary cognitive rehabilitation program for patients with mild Alzheimer's disease. Clinics (São Paulo, Brazil). 2011;**66**: 1395-1400. DOI: 10.1590/s1807-59322011000800015

[11] Bragin V. How to Activate Your Brain. Bloominton, IN: Authorhouse; 2007

[12] Dong H, Csernansky JG. Effects of stress and stress hormones on amyloid-beta protein and plaque deposition. Journal of Alzheimer's Disease. 2009;**18**(2):459-469. DOI: 10.3233/JAD-2009-1152

[13] Peers C, Dallas ML, Boycott HE, Scragg JL, Pearson HA, Boyle JP. Hypoxia and neurodegeneration. Annals of the New York Academy of Sciences. 2009;**1177**:169-177. DOI: 10.1111/j.1749-6632.2009.05026.x

[14] Wallace W, Ahlers ST, Gotlib J, Bragin V, Sugar J, Gluck R, et al. Amyloid precursor protein in the cerebral cortex is rapidly and persistently induced by loss of subcortical innervation. Proceedings of the National Academy of Sciences. 1993;**90**(18):8712-8716. DOI: 10.1073/pnas.90.18.8712

[15] Sabayan B, Jansen S, Oleksik AM, van Osch MJ, van Buchem MA, van Vliet P, et al. Cerebrovascular hemodynamics in Alzheimer's disease and vascular dementia: a meta-analysis of transcranial Doppler studies. Faseb Journal. 2011;**25**(1):5-13. DOI: 10.1096/fj.11-0102ufm

[16] Herholz K, Carter SF, Jones M. Positron emission tomography imaging

in dementia. The British Journal of Radiology. 2007;**80**(2):S160-S167. DOI: 10.1259/bjr/97295129

[17] Maksimovich IV. Vascular factors in Alzheimer's disease health. International Psychogeriatrics. 2012;**4**(Special Issue I):735-742. DOI: 10.4236/health.2012. 429114

[18] Sundström T, Elgh E, Larsson A, Näsman B, Nyberg L, Riklund KA. Memory-provoked rCBF-SPECT as a diagnostic tool in Alzheimer's disease? European Journal of Nuclear Medicine and Molecular Imaging. 2006;**33**(1):73-80. DOI: 10.1007/s00259-005-1874-0

[19] Nagahama Y, Nabatame H, Okina T, Yamauchi H, Narita M, Fujimoto N, et al. Cerebral correlates of the progression rate of the cognitive decline in probable Alzheimer's disease. European Neurology. 2003;**50**(1):1-9. DOI: 10.1159/000070851

[20] Silverman DH, Mosconi L, Ercoli L, Chen W, Small GW. Positron emission tomography scans obtained for the evaluation of cognitive dysfunction. Seminars in Nuclear Medicine. 2008;**38**(4):251-261. DOI: 10.1053/j.semnuclmed.2008.02.006

[21] Mehta L, Thomas S. The role of PET in dementia diagnosis and treatment. Applied Radiology. 2012;**41**(5):8-13

[22] van Halteren-van Tilborg IA, Scherder EJ, Hulstijn W. Motor-skill learning in Alzheimer's disease: A review with an eye to the clinical practice. Neuropsychology Review. 2007;**17**(3):203-212. DOI: 10.1007/s11065-007-9030-1

[23] Grady CL, Haxby JV, Horwitz B, Gillette J, Salerno JA, Gonzalez-Aviles A, et al. Activation of cerebral blood flow during a visuoperceptual task in patients with Alzheimer-type dementia.

Neurobiology of Aging. 1993;**14**(1):35-44. DOI: 10.1016/0197-4580(93)90018-7

[24] Cantón-Habas V, Rich-Ruiz M, Romero-Saldaña M, Carrera-González MDP. Depression as a risk factor for dementia and Alzheimer's disease. Biomedicine. 2020;**8**(11):457. DOI: 10.3390/biomedicines8110457

[25] Dumurgier J, Artaud F, Touraine C, Rouaud O, Tavernier B, Dufouil C, et al. Gait speed and decline in gait speed as predictors of incident dementia. The Journals of Gerontology. Series A, Biological Sciences and Medical Sciences. 2017;**72**(5):655-661. DOI: 10.1093/gerona/glw110

[26] Liou WC, Chan L, Hong CT, Chi WC, Yen CF, Liao HF, et al. Hand fine motor skill disability correlates with dementia severity. Archives of Gerontology and Geriatrics. 2020;**90**: 104168. DOI: 10.1016/j.archger. 2020.104168

[27] Selye H. Stress and the general adaptation syndrome. British Medical Journal. 1950;**1**(4667):1383-1392. DOI: 10.1136/bmj.1.4667.1383

[28] Nicholas J. Justice the relationship between stress and Alzheimer's disease. Neurobiology Stress. 2018;**8**:127-133. DOI: 10.1016/j.ynstr.2018.04.002

[29] Guerry MP, Jacobson MW, Salmon DP, Gamst AC, Patterson TL, Goldman S, et al. The influence of chronic stress on dementia-related diagnostic change in older adults. Alzheimer Disease and Associated Disorders. 2012;**26**(3):260-266. DOI: 10.1097/WAD.0b013e3182389a9c

[30] Sänger J, Bechtold L, Schoofs D, Blaszkewicz M, Wascher E. The influence of acute stress on attention mechanisms and its electrophysiological correlates. Frontiers in Behavioral Neuroscience. 2014;**8**:353. DOI: 10.3389/fnbeh.2014.00353

[31] Sandi C. Stress and cognition. Wiley Interdisciplinary Reviews: Cognitive Science. 2013;**4**(3):245-261. DOI: 10.1002/wcs.1222

[32] Stacey BS, Graham-Engeland JE, Engeland CG, Smyth JM, Almeida DM, Katz MJ, et al. The Effects of Stress on Cognitive Aging, Physiology and Emotion (ESCAPE) Project. BMC Psychiatry. 2015;**15**:1-14. DOI: 10.1186/s12888-015-0497-7

[33] Ávila-Villanueva M, Gómez-Ramírez J, Maestú F, Venero C, Ávila J, Fernández-Blázquez MA. The role of chronic stress as a trigger for the alzheimer disease continuum. Frontiers in Aging Neuroscience. 2020;**12**:561504. DOI: 10.3389/fnagi.2020.561504

[34] Liu YZ, Wang YX, Jiang CL. Inflammation: The common pathway of stress-related diseases. Frontiers in Human Neuroscience. 2017, 2017;**11**:316. DOI: 10.3389/fnhum.2017.00316

[35] Vedhara K, Hyde J, Gilchrist ID, Tytherleigh M, Plummer S. Acute stress, memory, attention and cortisol. Psychoneuroendocrinology. 2000;**25**(6): 535-549. DOI: 10.1016/s0306-4530(00)00008-1

[36] Stoia DCM, Ștefănuț A, Moldovan R, Hogea L, Giurgi-Oncu C, Bredicean C. Effectiveness of family stress-relief interventions for patients with dementia: A systematic evaluation of literature. Neuropsychiatric Disease and Treatment. 2020;**16**:629-635. DOI: 10.2147/NDT.S241150

[37] Stella F, Canonici AP, Gobbi S, Santos-Galduroz RF, de Castilho Cação J, Gobbi LTB, et al. Attenuation of neuropsychiatric symptoms and caregiver burden in Alzheimer's disease by motor intervention: A controlled trial. Clinics (Sao Paulo). 2011;**66**(8):1353-1360. DOI: 10.1590/S1807-59322011000800008

[38] Alexopoulos GS, Meyers BS, Young RC, Campbell S, Silbersweig D, Charlson M. 'Vascular depression' hypothesis. Archieves of General Psychiatry. 1997;**54**(10):915-922. DOI: 10.1001/archpsyc.1997.01830220033006

[39] Taylor WD, Aizenstein HJ, Alexopoulos GS. The vascular depression hypothesis: mechanisms linking vascular disease with depression. Molecular Psychiatry. 2013;**18**(9):963-974. DOI: 10.1038/mp.2013.20

[40] Christos GT, Siarkos KT, Politis AM. Unmet needs in pharmacological treatment of apathy in Alzheimer's disease: A systematic review. Frontiers in Pharmacology. 2019;**10**:1108. DOI: 10.3389/fphar.2019.01108

[41] Brodaty H. Burns K, Nonpharmacological management of apathy in dementia: A systematic review. The American Journal of Geriatric Psychiatry. 2012;**20**(7): 549-564. DOI: 10.1097/JGP.0b013e31822be242

[42] Theleritis C, Siarkos K, Politis AA, Katirtzoglou E. A systematic review of non-pharmacological treatments for apathy in dementia. International Journal of Geriatric Psychiatry. 2018;**33**(2):e177-e192. DOI: 10.1002/gps.4783

[43] Santabárbara J, Lipnicki DM, Bueno-Notivol J, Olaya-Guzmán B, Villagrasa B, López-Antón R. Updating the evidence for an association between anxiety and risk of Alzheimer's disease: A meta-analysis of prospective cohort studies. Journal of Affective Disorders. 2020;**262**:397-404. DOI: 10.1016/j.jad.2019.11.065

[44] Iadecola C. The overlap between neurodegenerative and vascular factors in the pathogenesis of dementia. Acta

Neuropathologica. 2010;**120**(3):287-296. DOI: 10.1007/s00401-010-0718-6

[45] Marchesi VT. Alzheimer's dementia begins as a disease of small blood vessels, damaged by oxidative-induced inflammation and dysregulated amyloid metabolism: Implications for early detection and therapy. Ageing Research Reviews. 2012;**11**(2):271-277. DOI: 10.1016/j.arr.2011.12.009

[46] Mazza M et al. Primary cerebral blood flow deficiency and Alzheimer's disease: Shadows and lights. Journal of Alzheimer's Disease. 2011;**23**(3):375-389. DOI: 10.3233/JAD-2010-090700

[47] Stafstrom CE, Rho JM. The ketogenic diet as a treatment paradigm for diverse neurological disorders. Frontiers in Pharmacology. 2012;**59**:1-5. DOI: 10.3389/fphar.2012.00059

[48] Remington R, Chan A, Paskavitz J, Shea TB. Efficacy of a vitamin/nutriceutical formulation for moderate-stage to later-stage Alzheimer's disease: A placebo-controlled pilot study. American Journal of Alzheimer's Disease and Other Dementias. 2009;**24**(1):27-33. DOI: 10.1177/1533317508325094

[49] Kamphuis PJ, Wurtman RJ. Nutrition and Alzheimer's disease: pre-clinical concepts. European Journal of Neurology. 2009;**16**(Suppl 1):12-18. DOI: 10.1111/j.1468-1331.2009.02737.x

[50] Shea TB, Rogers E, Remington R. Nutrition and dementia: Are we asking the right questions? Journal of Alzheimer's Disease. 2012;**30**(1):27-33. DOI: 10.3233/JAD-2012-112231

[51] Gillette-Guyonnet S, Nourhashemi F, Andrieu S, de Glisezinski I, Ousset PJ, Riviere D, et al. Weight loss in Alzheimer disease. The American Journal of Clinical Nutrition. 2000;**71**(2):637S-642S. DOI: 10.1093/ajcn/71.2.637s

[52] Herzig KH, Purhonen AK, Räsänen KM, Idziak J, Juvonen P, Phillps R, et al. Fecal pancreatic elastase-1 levels in older individuals without known gastrointestinal diseases or diabetes mellitus. BMC Geriatrics. 2011;**11**:4. DOI: 10.1186/1471-2318-11-4

[53] Hardt PD, Ewald N. Exocrine pancreatic insufficiency in diabetes mellitus: a complication of diabetic neuropathy or a different type of diabetes? Experimental Diabetes Research. 2011;**2011**:761950. DOI: 10.1155/2011/761950

[54] Mowat AMI. Historical Perspective: Metchnikoff and the intestinal microbiome. Journal of Leukocyte Biology. 2021;**109**(3):513-517. DOI: 10.1002/JLB.4RI0920-599

[55] Jenifer FK, Hillesheim E, Pereira ACSN, Camargo CQ, Rabito EI. Probiotics for dementia: A systematic review and meta-analysis of randomized controlled trials. Nutrition Reviews. 2021;**79**(2):160-170. DOI: 10.1093/nutrit/nuaa037

[56] Chudzik A, Orzyłowska A, Rola R, Stanisz GJ. Probiotics, prebiotics and postbiotics on mitigation of depression symptoms: modulation of the brain–gut–microbiome axis. Biomolecules. 2021;**11**(7):1000. DOI: 10.3390/biom11071000

[57] Philip AM. Recycling metchnikoff: Probiotics, the intestinal microbiome and the quest for long life. Frontiers in Public Health. 2013;**1**:52. DOI: 10.3389/fpubh.2013.00052

[58] Mozolic JL, Hayasaka S, Laurienti PJ. A cognitive training intervention increases resting cerebral blood flow in healthy older adults. Frontiers in Human Neuroscience. 2010;**4**(16):1-10. DOI: 10.3389/neuro.09.016.2010

[59] Kawashima R. Mental exercises for cognitive function: Clinical evidence.

Journal of Preventive Medicine and Public Health. 2013;**46**(Suppl 1):S22-S27. DOI: 10.3961/jpmph.2013.46.S.S22

[60] Lautenschlager NT, Cox KL, Flicker L, Foster JK, van Bockxmeer FM, Xiao J, et al. Effect of physical activity on cognitive function in older adults at risk for Alzheimer disease: A randomized trial. Journal of the American Medical Association. 2008;**300**(9):1027-1037. DOI: 10.1001/jama.300.9.1027

[61] Ahlskog JE, Geda YE, Graff-Radford NR, Petersen RC. Physical exercise as a preventive or disease-modifying treatment of dementia and brain aging. Mayo Clinic Proceedings. 2011;**86**(9):876-884. DOI: 10.4065/mcp.2011.0252

[62] Voigt RM et al. Systemic brain derived neurotrophic factor but not intestinal barrier integrity is associated with cognitive decline and incident Alzheimer's disease. PLoS One. 2021. DOI: 10.1371/journal.pone.0240342

[63] Sama FS et al. Exercise promotes the expression of brain derived neurotrophic factor (BDNF) through the action of the ketone body β-hydroxybutyrate. eLife. 2016;**5**: e15092. DOI: 10.7554/eLife15092

[64] Roland PE, Meyer E, Shibasaki T, Yamamoto YL, Thompson CJ. Regional cerebral blood flow changes in cortex and basal ganglia during voluntary movements in normal human volunteers. Journal of Neurophysiology. 1982;**48**(2):467-480. DOI: 10.1152/jn.1982.48.2.467

[65] Khalsa DS, Amen D, Hanks C, Money N, Newberg A. Cerebral blood flow changes during chanting meditation. Nuclear Medicine Communications. 2009;**30**(12):956-961. DOI: 10.1097/MNM.0b013e32832fa26c

[66] Deslandes A, Moraes H, Ferreira C, Veiga H, Silveira H, Mouta R, et al.

Exercise and mental health: many reasons to move. Neuropsychobiology. 2009;**59**:191-198. DOI: 10.1159/000223730

[67] Bragin V, Chemodanova M, Bragin I, Dzhafarova N, Mescher I, Chernyavskyy PE, et al. A 60-month follow-up of a naturalistic study of integrative treatment for real-life geriatric patients with depression, dementia and multiple chronic illnesses. Open Journal of Psychiatry. 2012;**2**:129-140

[68] Bragin V, Shereshevsky G, Gorskaya A, Dorfman E, Bragin I, Copeli F, et al. Arresting of cognitive decline for 72 months: a novel rehabilitation program for Alzheimer's dementia, based on pathogenesis of Alzheimer's disease and multiple intervention modalities. Copenhagen, Denmark: Alzheimer's Association International Conference; 2014

[69] Aliev G, Palacios HH, Lipsitt AE, Fischbach K, Lamb BT, Obrenovich ME, et al. Nitric oxide as an initiator of brain lesions during the development of Alzheimer disease. Neurotoxicity Research. 2009;**16**:293-305. DOI: 10.1007/s12640-009-9066-5

[70] Henry-Feugeas MC. Assessing cerebrovascular contribution to late dementia of the Alzheimer's type: the role of combined hemodynamic and structural MR analysis. Journal of the Neurological Sciences. 2009;**283**:44-48. DOI: 10.1016/j.jns.2009.02.325

[71] Zhang X, Le W. Pathological role of hypoxia in Alzheimer's disease. Experimental Neurology. 2010;**223**: 299-303. DOI: 10.1016/j.expneurol.2009.07.033

[72] Donev R, Kolev M, Millet B, Thome J. Neuronal death in Alzheimer's disease and therapeutic opportunities. Journal of Cellular and Molecular Medicine. 2009;**13**:4329-4348. DOI: 10.1111/j.1582-4934.2009.00889.x

[73] Heyn P. The effect of a multisensory exercise program on engagement, behavior, and selected physiological indexes in persons with dementia. American Journal of Alzheimer's Disease and Other Dementias. 2003;**18**:247-251. DOI: 10.1177/153331750301800409

[74] van Halteren-van Tilborg IA, Scherder EJ, Hulstijn W. Motor-skill learning in Alzheimer's disease: A review with an eye to the clinical practice. Neuropsychology Review. 2007;**17**:203-212. DOI: 10.1007/s11065-007-9030-1

[75] Gitlin LN, Winter L, Vause Earland T, Adel Herge E, Chernett NL, Piersol CV, et al. The tailored activity program to reduce behavioral symptoms in individuals with dementia: Feasibility, acceptability, and replication potential. Gerontologist. 2009;**49**:428-439.40. DOI: 10.1093/geront/gnp087

[76] Pitkala KH, Raivio MM, Laakkonen ML, Tilvis RS, Kautiainen H, Strandberg TE. Exercise rehabilitation on home-dwelling patients with Alzheimer's disease—a randomized, controlled trial. Study protocol. Trials. 2010;**11**:92. DOI: 10.1186/1745-6215-11-92

Chapter 3

# Alzheimer's Disease: An Insightful Review on the Future Trends of the Effective Therapeutics

*Afreen Hashmi, Vivek Srivastava, Syed Abul Kalam and Devesh Kumar Mishra*

## Abstract

Alzheimer's disease (AD) is a disorder of brain which progressively weakens the cognitive function. It is occur due to formation of β-amyloid plaques, neurofibrillary tangles, and degeneration of cholinergic neurotransmitter. There is no effective treatment capable of slowing down disease progression, current pharmacotherapy for AD only provides symptomatic relief and limited improvement in cognitive functions. Many molecules have been explored that show promising outcomes in AD therapy and can regulate cellular survival through different pathways. Present study involves current directions in the search for novel, potentially effective agents for the treatment of AD, as well as selected promising treatment strategies. These include agents acting upon the β-amyloid, such as vaccines, antibodies and inhibitors or modulators of γ- and β-secretase; agents directed against the tau protein. Current clinical trials with Aβ antibodies (solanezumab, bapineuzumab, and crenezumab) seem to be promising, while vaccines against the tau protein (AADvac1) are now in primary-stage trials. Most phase II clinical trials ending with a positive result do not succeed in phase III, often due to serious side effects or lack of therapeutic efficacy but Abucanumab (marketed as Aduhelm) now approved by USFDA in 2021 for the treatment of AD.

**Keywords:** neurodegeneration, novel strategies, clinical trials, medicinal plants

## 1. Introduction

Alzheimer's disease (AD) is a brain disorder described in 1906 by Aloes Alzheimer, a German physician [1]. It is a progressive and neurodegenerative disorder which mainly occur in old aged people of over 65 years of age [1–3]. For progression and development of disease various pathways are involved such as formation of plaque, inflammatory cascade, cholinergic deficit, oxidative stress, and many more. Senile plaques formation and neurofibrillary tangles persist significant neuro-pathological symbols of this disease. Senile plaques are the main component of amyloid beta (Aβ) peptide that are covered by dystrophic neurites and activated microglia. Accumulation of Aβ results changed process of proteolytic amyloid precursor protein (APP) through beta and gamma secretase. The β-amyloid peptide, with 39–42 amino acid residues (BAP), perform vital role in development of AD.

There are mainly two types of AD, familial AD which affects the people who have age less than 65. The other type of AD is sporadic AD which affect the people older than 65. At present there is no cure for Alzheimer's disease but it could me managed to some level by using available medications (**Table 1**) [6, 7].

## 1.1 Epidemiology

In 2020 approx. 50 million individual dealing with dementia worldwide. In India more than four million of people suffering from AD and dementia while in USA approx. 5.8 million living with dementia and AD. It is estimated that it is the fifth main source of death in USA and the number of death increased 146% between 2000 and 2018. It is predicted the causality will increase to 13.8 million which number of patient increases to 13.5 million by 2050. Elderly persons are more prone to younger one [8].

## 1.2 Etiology

In maximum case genetic lifestyle choices aging stress and environmental factors induces AD [9].

### 1.2.1 Age

Researchers have claimed that older adults have more risk of having AD. Scientists are still learning, how age-related changes in the brain may harm neurons and contribute to Alzheimer's [10].

### 1.2.2 Genetic factors

### 1.2.2.1 Early onset

It occur due to mutation in chromosome 1, 14, and 21. The changes on chromosome 1 produces PRESENILIN-2 (PSEN2) named protein while chromosome 14 produces PRESENILIN-1 (PSEN1). These PSEN 1 and PSEN 2 directly and indirectly both trigger/encode for membrane protein convoluted for amyloid precursor protein. These mutations reduce the effectiveness of γ-secretase, an enzyme which is responsible for formation of beta amyloid peptide (βAP) [11]. Amyloid precursor protein is

| Factors | Dementia | Alzheimer's disease | Normal aging |
|---|---|---|---|
| Definition | CNS disorder due to disease or any other pathological condition. | Common form of dementia. | Condition occur due to programmed cell death with time (gene therapy) and causes various disability. |
| Cause | AD, stroke, thyroid issues, vitamin deficiency, etc. | Deposition of beta amyloid protein in brain. | May cause biological systems to fail (DNA oxidation, DNA methylation, and apoptosis). |
| Duration and age | Permanent damage and 65 years and olders. | Average 8–20 years and 65 year but can occur as early as 30s. | Gradual and progressive condition until death. |
| Symptoms | Issues with memory, poor judgment, less focus and attention. | Difficulty to remembering newly learned information. | Bone break more easily, decrease overall energy, greater risk of heart stroke or hypothermia. |

**Table 1.**
*Alzheimer's disease versus dementia and normal aging [4, 5].*

coded on chromosome 21 and this mutation results in overproduction of beta amyloid peptide. Mutation on chromosome 1, 14, and 21 results in early onset AD [12].

### 1.2.2.2 Late onset

Apo-lipoprotein E (APOE) gene is responsible for late onset AD. APOE gene is lipid metabolism regulator which have an affinity for beta amyloid protein and increases the risk of AD. Chromosome 19 produces APOE gene. The inheritance of APOEe4 allele own genetic risk in sporadic AD. APOEe4 allele, age elevate the risk for development of late AD by two to three folds and two copies of five folds [13].

Variations in gene for receptor sortilin, SORT1, that is important for transferring APP from surface of cell to Golgi-endoplasmic reticulum complex, have been found in familial and sporadic types of AD [14].

### 1.2.2.3 Environmental factors

Conditions such as heart disease, stroke, high blood pressure, diabetes, and obesity are also linked as risk factors for AD [15].

## 2. Pathogenesis and clinical findings

The real origin of this disease is not well known but problems are linked with brain protein that work abnormally and cause malfunction. As a result neurons were damaged then fail to connect other neuron as a result they die. Initially the degradation starts within the region of brain which control memory ultimately dementia occur (**Figure 1**) [17].

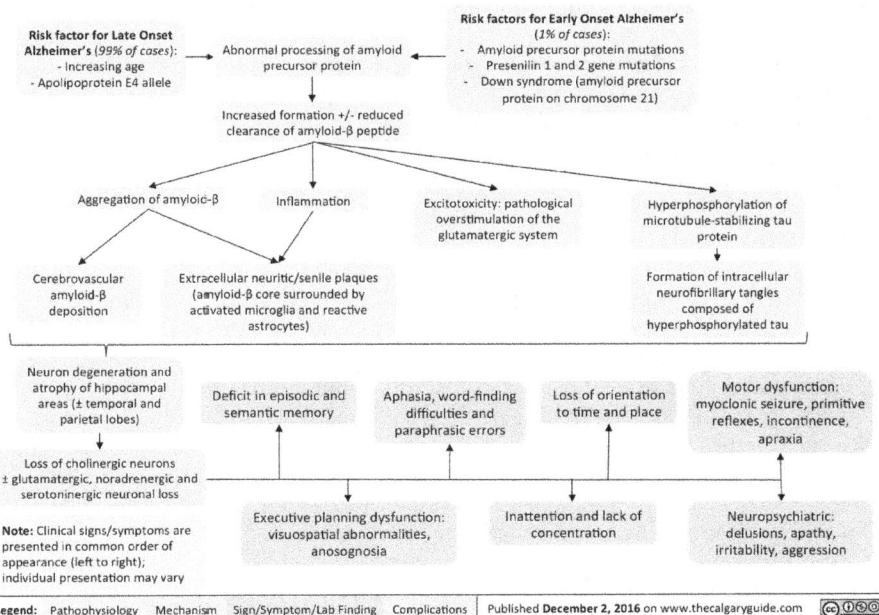

**Figure 1.**
*Clinical findings in Alzheimer's disease [16].*

## 2.1 Beta-amyloid protein aggregation and deposition

In the initial stage of AD amyloid proteins works abnormally and cause overproduction of beta amyloid secretase named enzyme split amyloid processor protein and due to deviation from this process, especially sudden change in gamma and beta secretases leads to unnatural production of amyloid beta [18].

## 2.2 Neurofibrillary hypothesis

Tau protein is known for its stabilizing property. It is useful in the transportation of nutrients and others essential matter within the neurons while in AD. Tau protein cause mutation and changes its structure which is known as neurofibrillary tangles [18, 19].

## 2.3 Cholinergic hypothesis

It is observed in the patient of AD there is deficiency of ACh due to abnormal functioning of choline acetyl transferase. This will treat as a clinical hallmark to support cholinergic hypothesis there is also a possible treatment of AD by increasing the level of ACh by reducing the activity of AChE cholinergic depletion observed after neurodegenerative cascade various cholinesterase inhibitors currently used in the treatment of AD [20].

## 2.4 Excitotoxicity

It is defined as the excess interaction of neurotransmitter glutamate and other excitatory neurotransmitter which may act as a potent neurotoxins for Alzheimer [21].

## 2.5 Vascular diseases and high cholesterol

Apo-lipoprotein E play important role in the cholesterol transportation and catabolism of triglyceride lipoprotein. Cholesterol also alter the clearance of amyloid beta and generation of NFT in neuronal membrane APOE4 also enhance the deposition of beta amyloid protein. High level of cholesterol in brain there by alter the member functioning this leads to plaque formation resulting AD [22].

## 2.6 Oxidative stress

Oxidative stress is generated due to imbalance of ROS generation and its quenching. Brain is more prone for oxidative stress due to high consumption of $O_2$. High level of polyunsaturated fatty acid. Low level of antioxidants and high level of redox transition metal ions. These all factors facilitate the production of reactive oxygen species like superoxide, hydrogen peroxide, etc. These ROS interact with surroundings proteins nucleic acids, etc. and cause cellular dysfunction [23]. There is also a close relationship between amyloid beta and oxidative stress because amyloid beta elevate the formation of ROS and initiate mitochondrial damage. This will also cause oxidative damage. These effects can also be observed in brain of triple transgenic mouse model of AD where tocopherol and GSH level decrease while lipid peroxidation is increased [24]. However this was observed before any plaque formation. While in another model dual mutant APP was expressed, oxidative stress and inflammation was induced by thiamine deficiency provoke plaque formation and enhance the level of amyloid [25].

## 2.7 Mitochondrial dysfunction

It is observed in the marphotric analysis of AD patients brain showed significant deficiency of mitochondria while its DNA and protein concentration elevate in cytoplasm and in the vacuoles associated with lipofuscin [26]. These mitochondria may be damaged due to autophagy and oxidative stress. Mitochondrial cytochrome oxidase activity also reduced in cortical region of AD brain. Due to this deficiency mitochondrial dysfunction occur and ROS generated and energy stores were decreased and ultimately neurodegeneration occur [27].

## 2.8 Inflammatory mediators

Amyloid deposition in brain also associated with local inflammation and immunologic alleviations [28]. This association induces the release of $NO_3$, cytokines which cause neural damage and cause inflammation [29, 30].

## 3. Role of sex hormone in Alzheimer's

Evidence from animal and human studies support functional roles of sex hormones like estrogens, progesterone, and androgens in behavior and cognition. With several neuroprotective activity involved, age reduces level of sex hormones were connected with greater possibilities of cognitive degeneration and AD. For example, in females development of AD is associated with decreased exposure to estrogens across the lifetime, while in males age related degeneration in both levels of peripheral and brain testosterone is linked with greater susceptibilities of AD development. Also, alterations in receptors of sex hormone and downstream signaling pathways during aging have been stated. For example, the nonfunctional splicing estrogen variants receptor alpha in the hippocampus was enhanced throughout aging and AD, with advanced levels in female old age subjects in comparison to males. Moreover, studies recognized polymorphisms of estrogen receptors related with intellectual decay and AD development in females, especially in APOE ε4 (APOE4) transporters. These information recommended diminished responsiveness of brain to sex hormones during aging and disease development. However, clinical trial outcomes of sex hormone therapy in AD are rather contentious. Despite prior studies associating protective activity of estrogen replacement against AD in females, huge clinical studies failed to exhibit any useful possessions. It was suggested that replacement of hormone initiation in the serious window of perimenopause may diminish the risks of dementia, while it might raise the risks if started a very long time after menopause. Moreover treatment timing, reduced responsiveness at receptors of brain and downstream signaling pathways might add to the uselessness of hormonal therapy. Together, these investigations recommend the complication of sex hormones association in AD [31].

## 4. Strategies used in the treatment of Alzheimer's disease: A clinical data

### 4.1 Conventional approaches

Currently there is no cure for this disease, the objective of several medicine is used to reduce symptoms linked with disease and to reduce disease progression (**Table 2**) [32–36].

| Drug name | Indication | Mode of action | Adverse effect |
|---|---|---|---|
| Donepezil | Minor to chronic | It stops the breakdown of ACh by preventing the function of acetyl cholinesterase | Fatigue, abnormal dreams, hallucinations, confusion, hypertension, abdominal pain |
| | | Treats intellectual indication of AD | |
| Galantamine | Minor to medium | Stops the breakdown of Ach and stimulates receptors to discharge extra ACh | Somnolence, bradycardia, insomnia, urinary tract infection, anorexia, syncope |
| | | Treats intellectual indication of AD | |
| Rivastigmine | Minor to medium | Stops the breakdown of Ach by preventing the enzymes that abolish ACh | Dizziness, diarrhea, anxiety, vertigo, asthenia, tachycardia |
| | Also used to treat dementia from Parkinson's disease | Treats intellectual indication of AD | |
| Memantine | Medium to severe | Blocks glutamatergic (NMDA) receptors and controls the action of glutamate | Headache, constipation, vomiting, backache |
| | | Treats intellectual indication of AD | |
| Donepezil/memantine | Medium to severe | it binds to NMDA receptor-operated caption channels, and gives therapeutic effects by preventing persistent stimulation in CNS | Hallucination, headache, cough, fatigue, cramping, syncope, increased frequency of bowel movements |

**Table 2.**
*Currently used drug for the treatment of Alzheimer's disease.*

## 4.2 Current scenario

### 4.2.1 Antiamyloidogenic pathway and amyloidogenic route as approaches for development of therapeutic treatments adjusting the course of Alzheimer's disease

From the previous eras, the pharmaceutical industry has decided to chiefly focused on the amyloidocentric method, dedicating significant possessions to form useful AD drugs. Nevertheless, numerous failures of drug candidates in clinical trials have led investigators to question the viability of this approach [10–12]. Possible cause for failure is a absence of biomarkers that could consistently recognize AD in comparatively initial phases. It is totally promising that the patients presently enrolled for phase III trials are in such advanced phases of AD that any attempted interference is possibly inadequate. In the meantime, there is still a number of new management under development, that focused the amyloidogenic route. In order to decrease generation of Aβ from the APP, inhibition of γ- and β-secretase and the potentiation of activity of α-secretase have been deliberated.

### 4.2.2 Inhibitors and modulators of β-secretase

β-secretase enzyme complex contributes in the primary phases of the amyloidogenic APP-processing pathway. The inhibitors of β-secretase development is a task because, besides the APP, this complex has several substrates. To give just one example, neuregulin-1, that included in the CNS axons myelination and synaptic elasticity, is a target β-secretase. Substrates wide range results to substantial adverse effects, even if the precise enzyme inhibition is reached. But, E2609 (clinical trial ID# NCT01600859), MK-8931 (NCT01739348), and LY2886721 (NCT01807026 and NCT01561430) have all exposed efficiency in decreasing the production of Aβ by up to 80–90% in the cerebrospinal fluid (CSF) in humans. None of inhibitors of β-secretase have touched the market so far [37–40].

### 4.2.3 Inhibitors and modulators of γ-secretase

In the final stage of amyloidogenesis, γ-secretase complex is responsible for the production of Aβ(1–40) and Aβ(1–42). Inhibition of γ-secretase was firstly proposed strategy for the management of Alzheimer's disease but the substrate promiscuity shows equal issues facing γ-secretase inhibitors. γ-secretase proposed to target the Notch protein which is responsible for the regulation of cell proliferation, development, differentiation and cellular communication but off target secondary effects are major concern [41–43].

Semagacestat (LY450139) named γ-secretase inhibitor reduces the Aβ level in the blood and in cerebrospinal fluid [44]. The results obtained from the clinical study conducted on 3000 patients shows the major adverse effects like decrease cognition abilities and difficulty in the carry out daily living activities and elevated skin cancer incidence and increased risk of infection and weight loss. Another γ-secretase named avagacestat discontinued in the development stage due to lack of efficacy (NCT00810147, NCT00890890, NCT00810147, NCT01079819, [45–47]).

Several nonsteroidal anti-inflammatory drugs like indomethacin, ibuprofen, flurbiprofen, sulindac also decreases the Aβ(1–42) peptide levels in in-vivo and in in-vitro studies. Ibuprofen is a cyclooxigenase inhibitor while R-flurbiprofen (tarenflurbil) is not, so the reduction of Aβ(1–42) peptide levels is not associated with the COX inhibition. Unfortunately, in clinical trials tarenflurbil and ibuprofen does not shows efficacy for the treatment of Alzheimer's disease. The idea of long term use of NSAID's for the treatments of Alzheimer's disease as NSAIDS reduces the Aβ peptide level in blood but negative results reported in the clinical studies that's why this hypothesis requires further investigations [48, 49].

Clinical studies with 8-hydroxiquinolines compounds like clioquinol and PBT2 also conducted for the treatment of Alzheimer's disease. The mechanism of action is yet established, but the expected MOA suggested that the increased levels of oxidative stress is due to the copper ions binding to Aβ, leading to metal-mediated generation of ROS (reactive oxygen species). It is proposed that the 8-hydroxiquinolines may prevent Aβ aggregation and restoring homeostasis in the cellular levels of copper and zinc ions. But after in clinical development these compounds failed due to lack of efficacy [50–52].

### 4.2.4 Agents that stimulate the removal of amyloid deposits and aggregates

Another possible treatment choice that is involved on the amyloidogenic pathway is to stimulate the existing amyloid aggregates clearance. To achieve this, three different approaches have been assessed.

## 4.2.5 Activation of enzymes that destroy amyloid plaques

Amyloid plaques are destroyed by various proteases comprising neprilysin, IDE, plasmin, angiotensin converting enzyme, endothelin converting enzyme, and metalloproteinases. Levels of protein these enzymes reduces in AD, that promotes accumulation and formation of Aβ. Despite being an attractive approach for forming disease-modifying medicine, no compounds with this MOA have ever entered advanced clinical development because of lack of specificity.

## 4.2.6 Modulation of β-amyloid transport between the brain and the peripheral circulation

Transport of Aβ between the circulation of CNS and peripheral is controlled by: (i) apolipoproteins (e.g., Aβ might be transported from the blood to the brain when it is bound to APOE); (ii) low-density lipoprotein receptor-related protein (LRP-1), that enhances Aβ discharge from the brain to the blood; (iii) receptor for progressive glycation end products (RAGE), that enables the Aβ transport across the blood-brain barrier (BBB) [53, 54].

Any treatment goal, that is determined on this mechanism, is to decrease the load of cerebral amyloid by trying to control Aβ to the peripheral circulation. To this end, a different number of approaches have been suggested, particularly the administration of LRP-1 peripherally. Though, the only drug candidates that have entered the clinical phase are the RAGE inhibitors.

## 4.2.7 Antiamyloid immunotherapy

### 4.2.7.1 Active immunotherapy

Immunotherapy approach designed to stimulate clearance of Aβ with the aimed of decreasing load of amyloid load in AD. Active immunization (vaccination) with either Aβ(1–42) (main form found in senile plaques) or other synthetic fragments has been positively assessed in transgenic mouse models of AD. Human tests were primarily hopeful; though first-generation vaccine (AN1792) treatment has shown major adverse events which results to the phase II trials cessation. AN1792 contained of a synthetic full-length Aβ(1–42) peptide with a QS-21 adjuvant. Because of a T cell-mediated autoimmune response, 6% of patients have established inflammation in brain that ended up being aseptic meningoencephalitis [55].

Second-generation vaccines were planned utilizing a limited portion of Aβ(1–6) peptide in an try to inhibit nonspecific immune response seen with the full-length vaccine. Novartis designed CAD 106, was the first second-generation vaccine which moved to development phase. Newly finished phase II trial have exposed a Aβ-specific antibody response in 75% of treated patients, without producing any side effect. Janssen developed ACC-001, has freshly finished two-phase II trials (NCT01284387 and NCT00479557) with an additional phase II trial still continuing (NCT01227564). Though, the pharmaceutical industry has canceled the ideas for this vaccine development. Further vaccines, comprising tetra-palmitoylated Aβ(1–15) re-formed in a liposome (ACI-24), MER5101 and AF205 are now in different phases of preclinical progression [56–58].

### 4.2.7.2 Passive immunization

It is the monoclonal or polyclonal antibodies administration directed against Aβ. This treatment contains intravenous administration of anti-Aβ antibodies to the patient. The advantage of this approach is to match to active immunization is which the proinflammatory T cell-mediated immune response should not arise. Reports have shown that in transgenic animals passive immunization decreases the load of cerebral amyloid and recovers cognition, even when the amyloid plaque numbers are not suggestively decreased. This could be recognized to the soluble amyloid oligomers neutralization, that progressively identified to play an important role in the pathophysiology of AD.

Bapineuzumab and solanezumab are two monoclonal antibodies which are reach now present in advanced phase of development. Though, two phase III trials had failed in 2012 due to low effectiveness in patients with mild-to-moderate AD [59]. Both are humanized monoclonal antibodies against Aβ(1–6) and Aβ(12–28), respectively. In bapineuzumab, noteworthy decrease in brain amyloid plaques and phosphorylated Tau in cerebrospinal fluid was stated. Though, the treatment unsuccessful to give noteworthy developments of brain function. In a solanezumab trial, infusions of 400 mg of solanezumab or placebo were given for 80 weeks once a month in patients with mild-to-moderate AD. The outcomes recommended that solanezumab might recover cognition in mild AD; but statistical significance was not attained in study. Presently solanezumab present in phase III trials in patients with AD (NCT01127633 and NCT01900665) and in older persons who have common thinking and memory function but who might be at danger of AD developing in the future (NCT02008357, [60, 61]).

Crenezumab (MABT5102A) is a humanized monoclonal antibody that uses IgG4 backbone. In April 2014 a stage II trial to measure the safety and effectiveness in patients with mild-to-moderate AD (NCT01343966) was accomplished, while the outcomes are not yet openly accessible. The supreme stage II trial pointing to assess the safety and effectiveness of crenezumab in asymptomatic transporters of E280A autosomal-dominant mutation of PSEN1 initiated in November 2013 (NCT01998841).

Other monoclonal antibodies against Aβ established so far contain PF-04360365 (ponezumab) that targets the free carboxy terminal amino acids 33–40 of the Aβ peptide; MABT5102A, that binds to Aβ monomers, oligomers, and fibrils with similarly great affinity; GSK933776A, that is likewise to bapineuzumab in which it binds to the N-terminal Aβ(1–5). Additional, other passive immunotherapies typically in stage I clinical trial involve NI-101, SAR-228810, and BAN-2401 [58, 62].

### 4.2.8 Approaches focused on Tau proteins

In neurons Tau proteins are extremely soluble and abundant where they play a important role in stabilization of microtubule, mainly in axons [63]. Tau hyperphosphorylation resulting the insoluble paired helical filaments (PHF) development that form neurofibrillary tangles. The microtubule-binding capacity damage initiate destabilization of cytoskeleton, that ultimately develops neurodegeneration and neuronal death [64]. As a substitute to amyloidocentric strategies, this treatments goal to prevent the phosphorylation of Tau protein. Additional, microtubule-stabilizing drugs can be utilized as a disease-modifying approach in AD. In current years, immunomodulation was recommended as a feasible choice for stimulating operative Tau aggregates clearance [65].

### 4.2.9 Hyperphosphorylation of Tau inhibitors

All Tau proteins are a result of different splicing of a microtubule-associated protein Tau (MAPT) gene. Primary mechanism that controls Tau binding to microtubules is phosphorylation. The protein remains soluble under physiological circumstances; though, in this disease, pathological hyperphosphorylation of Tau compromises its regular functions [66, 67]. Imbalance between the catalytic activity of kinases and phosphatases occurs hyperphosphorylation. Enhanced expression of active forms of several kinases in the areas proximal to neurofibrillary tangles has been labeled in AD, comprising CDK5, GSK3β, Fyn, stress-activated protein kinases JNK and p38, and mitogen-activated protein kinases ERK1 and ERK2 [68]. Certain kinases promote continuation of tau phosphorylation in neurofibrillary tangles. Resulting, noteworthy research determinations have been dedicated to the kinase inhibitors development as a probable treatment approach for AD. For example, SP600125, a extensively utilized pan-JNK inhibitor, employs valuable effects on cognition and decreases neurodegeneration in an APP/PS1 transgenic mouse model of AD. It has been planned which precise inhibition of JNK3 can be adequate to carry comparable benefits as seen with SP600125 in rodent models. Human data in AD patients designate a positive correlation between the JNK3 and Aβ(1–42) levels in the brain. Moreover, JNK3 upregulation was distinguished in the CSF and was related with loss of memory. Consequently, inhibition of JNK3 remains a capable goal for future treatments [69–71].

### 4.2.10 Tau aggregation inhibitors

Tau hyperphosphorylation contribute to neurotoxicity detected in AD brain. Methylene blue dye derivatives have revealed certain potential Tau aggregates formation inhibition. Methylene blue disturbs the Tau aggregation, has the capability to prevent amyloid aggregation, recovers the effectiveness of mitochondrial electron transport chain, decreases oxidative stress, stops mitochondrial impairment, and is also an autophagy modulator. The first-generation molecule resulting from methylene blue (Rember) seemed to stabilize AD development in a clinical trial that continued 50 weeks. These outcomes encouraged investigators to form a next-generation form of methylene blue, TRx 0237. This agents is a purified derivative of methylene blue that not only prevents aggregation of Tau protein but also liquefies brain tau aggregates. Various trials are presently ongoing (NCT01626391, NCT01689233, NCT01689246, NCT01626378) to assess the possible effectiveness of this agent in AD [72, 73].

### 4.2.11 Stabilizers of microtubule

Stabilization of microtubule might possibly attain a comparable end-result as which seen with the Tau hyperphosphorylation inhibitors. Paclitaxel is a microtubule-stabilizing agents presently in utilize in the oncology arena. Inappropriately, this agents is unable of BBB crossing and its utilize is related with major adverse events, that limits its efficacy in AD. In addition to paclitaxel, other microtubule-stabilizing agents like TPI 287 have been measured as a probable AD remedy. TPI 287 is a derivative of taxane, also utilize in the treatment of cancer. TPI 287 alleviates the microtubules by binding to tubulin. NCT01966666 trial will estimate TPI-287 safety, pharmacokinetic possessions, and tolerability by intravenous infusion in mild-to-moderate AD.

Epothilone D is a microtubule-stabilizing agent that enhanced axonal transport, decrease axonal dystrophy, reduced Tau neuropathology, and decreased hippocampal loss of neuron; though, in 2013 drug development for AD was discontinued after an unsuccessful clinical trial. With respect to Tau, more research are essential in order to better understand the exact molecular mechanisms elaborate in neurotoxicity of Tau. Current research associating the neurotoxic profiles of different forms of Tau recommend which is a soluble form is probable the greatest toxic. Thus, future therapeutic approaches should be focused on aiming Tau soluble forms [74].

### 4.2.12 Anti-Tau immunotherapy

Just as with the immunotherapies aiming Aβ, both passive and active immunization approaches against Tau have been measured. It was established that decrease in formation of Tau aggregate and enhanced Tau oligomers clearance and insoluble aggregates could all be reached with either active or passive immunotherapies. In rodents, treatment with monoclonal antibodies directed against hyperphosphorylated Tau has results to improvements in cognition and was not connected with noteworthy side effects.

Axon neuroscience began a stage I trial in 2013 to estimate the safety and tolerability of AADvac-1, an active immunotherapy that contains synthetic peptide derived from the Tau sequence coupled to keyhole limpet hemocyanin; the precise molecular nature of the antigen has not been disclosed (NCT01850238 and NCT02031198). AADvac-1 uses aluminum hydroxide as an adjuvant. At the 2014 Alzheimer's Association International Conference (AAIC) in Copenhagen, good preclinical safety profile was reported for the treatment period of up to 6 months in rats, rabbits, and dogs. These initial outcomes are hopeful and it remains to be seen whether AADvac-1 will prove satisfactory safety and efficiency in patients [75, 76].

### 4.2.13 The cholinergic hypothesis

The hippocampus, the chief region of brain elaborate in memory processing, is influenced by modulation of cholinergic neurotransmitter. One of the well categorized irregularities linked with neurotransmitter deviations is the cholinergic neurons degeneration in the nucleus basalis of Meynert and the cholinergic inputs loss to the neocortex and hippocampus. Various studies reported reduced in choline acetyltransferase (ChAT), acetylcholine (ACh) release, as well as decreases in nicotinic and muscarinic receptors in the cerebral cortex and hippocampus of postmortem AD brains. Acetylcholinesterase inhibitors (AChEI), one of the only two classes of compounds that presently accepted for AD treatment, act by stimulating ACh bioavailability at the synapse. Inappropriately, none of these agents are proficient of withdrawing the course of AD nor of even noticeably reducing down the degree of disease development. Their clinical effect is basically palliative; though, their possible utilize in combination therapy with other disease-modifying agents should not be omitted [77, 78].

### 4.2.14 Altering the perception: AD as a metabolic disorder

As revealed by clinical study data and research articles that diabetes is a one of the key factor that leads to AD pathology and unfolds the close connection between insulin-deficient diabetes and cerebral amyloidosis. These data also suggests about insulin signaling impairments (both peripheral and central) is possibly be existing in both diseases. Hence, considering insulin hormone at the core, "type 3 diabetes" hypothesis of AD was developed, observing metabolic phenotypes into a coherent framework [79].

The most anticipated mechanisms for the development of AD due to diabetes could be: glucose toxicity, insulin resistance, oxidative stress, elevated levels of advanced glycation end products, and cytokine-mediated neuroinflammation. Recently, Clarke and colleagues demonstrated that neuroinflammatory cascades can be initiated by the administration of soluble hypothalamic Aβ oligomers that ultimately causes disturbances in peripheral glucose homeostasis. Tumor necrosis factor α (TNFα) may have a significant role during this process [80].

Rosiglitazone and pioglitazone are used as antidiabetic drugs, which regulate glucose homeostasis by increasing insulin sensitivity, reducing blood glucose levels, and improving lipid metabolism. Both compounds have also been studied as potential therapeutics for AD treatment, with reported improvements in mitochondrial oxidative metabolism [81]. In animal models, pioglitazone modified various indices of brain aging but did not slow down the cognitive decline. Rosiglitazone and pioglitazone also induce the expression of peroxisome proliferator-activated receptor-γ co-activator 1 alpha (PGC-1α), a molecule that plays multiple roles in mitochondrial biogenesis, energy metabolism, and mitochondrial antioxidants expression. Previous studies have demonstrated that, in the human brain tissues, the expression of PGC-1α decreases with progression of AD dementia. Thus, PGC-1α upregulation may improve the mitochondrial energy metabolism and AD pathology [82–86].

In a small scale clinical trial on mild-to-moderate AD patients, it was found that pioglitazone enhances memory and cognition. On the other hand clinical trial (phase II) with larger group of patients (who did not possess an ApoE4 allele) were on treatment with rosiglitazone (6 months) shows improvement in memory retention and attention. However, similar study (phase III trial) using rosiglitazone failed to show efficacy in AD (NCT00550420). It is important to note that rosiglitazone was administered at much lower dosage than required to exert efficacious effects on AD pathophysiology in these trials, in rodent models of the disease. NCT00348140 recently completed clinical trial in which rosiglitazone was administrated in combination with AChEIs in patients with AD (mild-to-moderate) and until now no further outcome yet reported.

As a treatment possibility for AD, intranasal insulin have also been considered as it bypasses the BBB easily; adding the advantage of possibly minimum adverse events in peripheral tissues. Theoretically it is well established that direct delivery of insulin to the brain will activate cerebral insulin signaling leading to enhancements in memory processing resulting into neuroprotection. A recent ongoing clinical trial (with NCT017679090 is assessing long-term (12 months) efficacy of intranasal insulin (Humulin R U-100) among mild AD patients [87].

Also, it has been found that reduced plasma amylin concentrations may contribute in the progression of AD. As revealed by transgenic animal models of AD, amylin and pramlintide (amylin analog) reduced the brain Aβ levels and advances cognition. Interestingly, amylin inhibits β-secretase, whereas pramlintide did not [88].

## 5. Medicinal plants for the treatment of Alzheimer's disease

Here is the number of herbal plants reported to might have anti-Alzheimer activity (**Table 3**).

## 6. Recent advances in the treatment of Alzheimer's disease

In 2021 USFDA approved **Aducanumab** (marketed as Aduhelm) for the treatment of Alzheimer's disease. It is an amyloid beta-directed antibody approved under the accelerated approval pathway based on reductioning amyloid β plaques observed in patients treated with this drug.

It was approved for medical use in the United States. Aducanumab has since been approved by the Ministry of Health and Prevention in the United Arab Emirates as of October 3, 2021, making it the second country in the world to approve the treatment.

**Pharmacology-Mechanism of Action:** Immunoglobulin gamma 1 (IgG1) monoclonal antibody directed against aggregated soluble and insoluble forms of

| Sr. No. | Work done | Plant used | Common name | Author | Year | Ref. |
|---|---|---|---|---|---|---|
| 1. | Effects of the hydroethanolic extract of *Lycopodium selago* L. on scopolamine-induced memory deficits in zebrafish | *L. selago* | Fir clubmoss | Valu et al. | 2021 | [89] |
| 2. | Evaluation of traditional herb extract *Salvia officinalis* in treatment of Alzheimer's disease | *S. officinalis* | Sage | Datta et al. | 2020 | [90] |
| 3. | Protective effects of tenuifolin isolated from *Polygala tenuifolia* Willd roots on neuronal apoptosis and learning and memory deficits in mice with Alzheimer's disease | *P. tenuifolia* | Yuan zhi | Wang et al. | 2019 | [91] |
| 4. | *Convolvulus pluricaulis* (Shankhapushpi) ameliorates human microtubule-associated protein tau (*hMAPτ*) induced neurotoxicity in Alzheimer's disease *Drosophila* model | *C. pluricaulis* | Shankhapushpi | Kizhakke et al. | 2019 | [92] |
| 5. | *Malva parviflora* extract ameliorates the deleterious effects of a high fat diet on the cognitive deficit in a mouse model of Alzheimer's disease by restoring microglial function via a PPAR-γ-dependent mechanism | *M. parviflora* | Cheeseweed | Jiménez et al. | 2019 | [93] |
| 6. | Antioxidant, anti-Alzheimer and anti-parkinson activity of *Artemisia nilagirica* leaves with flowering tops | *A. nilagirica* | Indian wormwood | Pal and Pradeep | 2018 | [94] |
| 7. | Antioxidant and anti-acetylcholinesterase activities of essential oils from garlic (*Allium sativum*) Bulbs | *A. sativum* | Garlic | Akinyemi et al. | 2018 | [95] |
| 8. | Nootropic activity of ethanolic extract of *Alangium salvifolium* leaves on scopolamine mouse model of Alzheimer's disease | *A. salvifolium* | Ankol | Parameshwari et al. | 2018 | [96] |

| Sr. No. | Work done | Plant used | Common name | Author | Year | Ref. |
|---|---|---|---|---|---|---|
| 9. | *Moringa oleifera* alleviates homocysteine-induced Alzheimer's disease-like pathology and cognitive impairment | *M. oleifera* | Drumstick tree | Mahaman et al. | 2018 | [97] |
| 10. | Ameliorative effect of *Cleome gynandra* L. against scopolamine induced amnesia in mice | *C. gynandra* | Shonna cabbage | Manasa et al. | 2017 | [98] |
| 11. | Evaluation of nootropic activity of green peas in mice | *Pisum sativum* | Green peas | Kaura et al. | 2017 | [99] |
| 12. | Ameliorative effect of *Apium graveolens* Linn on scopolamine-induced amnesia mice | *A. graveolens* | Celery | Phetcharat et al. | 2017 | [100] |
| 13. | Evaluation of effect of alcoholic extract of *Tinospora cordifolia* on learning and memory in alprazolam induced amnesia in albino mice | *T. cordifolia* | Guduchi | Jyothi et al. | 2016 | [101] |
| 14 | Effect of *Camellia sinensis* on spatial memory in a rat model of Alzheimer's disease | *C. sinensis* | Green tea | Mahmoodzadeh et al. | 2016 | [102] |
| 15. | Evaluation of nootropic activity of *Curcuma longa* leaves in diazepam and scopolamine-induced amnesic mice and rats | *C. longa* | Turmeric | Reddy et al. | 2015 | [103] |
| 16. | Effect of ethanolic seed extract of *Bauhinia purpurea* linn on cognition in scopolamine induced Alzheimer's disease rat's model | *B. purpurea* | Orchid tree | Nemalapalli et al. | 2015 | [104] |
| 17. | *Mori fructus* improves cognitive and neuronal dysfunction induced by beta-amyloid toxicity through the GSK-3β pathway in vitro and in vivo | *M. fructus* | Mora | Kim et al. | 2015 | [105] |
| 18. | Anticholinesterase and antioxidant properties of aqueous extract of *Cola acuminate* seed *in vitro* | *C. acuminate* | Cola nut | Oboh et al. | 2014 | [106] |

| Sr. No. | Work done | Plant used | Common name | Author | Year | Ref. |
|---|---|---|---|---|---|---|
| 19. | Antiamnesic effect of piracetam potentiated with *Emblica officinalis* and *C. longa* in aluminum induced neurotoxicty of Alzheimer's disease | *E. officinalis* | Aamla | Ramachandran et al. | 2013 | [107] |
| 20 | Antiamnesic activity of *Syzygium cumini* against scopolamine induced spatial memory impairments in rats | *S. cumini* | Jamun | Alikatte et al. | 2012 | [108] |
| 21 | Acetylcholine and memory-enhancing activity of *Ficus racemosa* bark | *F. racemosa* | Cluster fig | Faiyaz et al. | 2011 | [109] |
| 22 | Protective effect of *Morinda citrifolia* fruits on beta-amyloid (25–35) induced cognitive dysfunction in mice: an experimental and biochemical study | *M. citrifolia* | Noni | Muralidharan et al. | 2010 | [110] |

**Table 3.**
*Plants studied in Alzheimer's disease.*

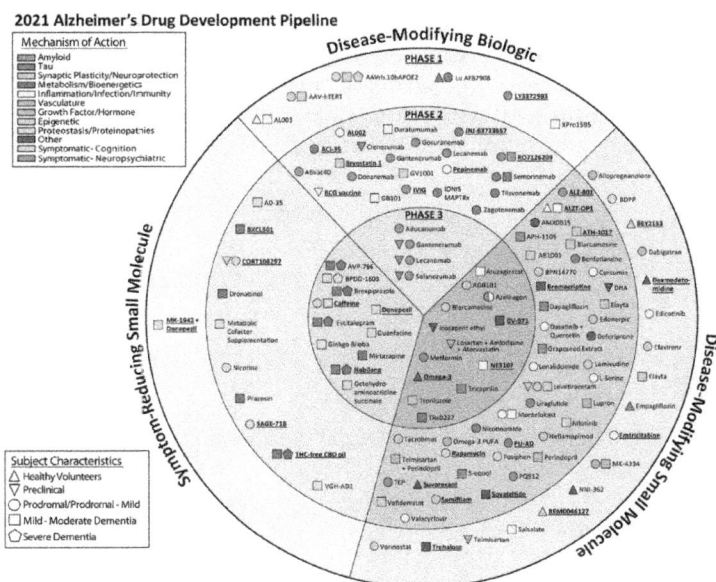

**Figure 2.**
*Drugs in clinical trials for treatment of Alzheimer's disease in 2021. In which the shape of icons shows the population involve in trials; the outer ring shows drugs in Phase I; the middle rings shows drugs in Phase II; the inner most ring shows drugs in Phase III trials [16].*

amyloid beta. The buildup of beta amyloid plaques in brain is crucial pathophysiological hallmark of Alzheimer's disease.

**Dosage Form and Strength:** Aduhelm is a clear to opalescent and colorless to yellow solution, accessible as: Injection: 170 mg/1.7 mL (100 mg/mL) in a single-dose vial and 300 mg/3 mL (100 mg/mL) in a single-dose vial [111].

**Who should take this drug?**

It is suggested for mild cognitive impairment (MCI) or mild dementia stage of Alzheimer's disease [112, 113].

### 6.1 Novel compound under investigation

Here is the figure that shows the agents which is in developing stage involve in the trials for the management of Alzheimer's disease. Most of agents in the trial target disease modification [114] (**Figure 2**).

In which the shape of icons shows the population involve in trials; the outer ring shows drugs in phase I; the middle rings shows drugs in phase II; the inner most ring shows drugs in phase III trials [115].

## 7. Conclusion

Alzheimer's disease is serious brain disorder, at present there is no cure for this disease but currently it can be controlled by using a drugs which symptomatically treat AD. AChE inhibitors are the first approved anti-AD drugs by the FDA, and they are also the first and the most useful drug used in the clinical treatment of AD. But now few of drugs also approved by USFDA in 2021 for the treatment of AD and few also in the trial phase. Results from clinical studies have shown different new drugs in pipeline and various novel approaches may also beneficial for treating AD. Interests in the utilization of different herbal products also increase day by day. This study provides the details about recent advancement the medicinal plants against the Alzheimer's disease. Availability of these new medicinal plants for AD will further increase the treatment options and thus provide a significant benefit to patients who remain uncontrollable to existing therapy.

## Author details

Afreen Hashmi*, Vivek Srivastava, Syed Abul Kalam and Devesh Kumar Mishra
Amity Institute of Pharmacy, Amity University Uttar Pradesh, Lucknow, India

*Address all correspondence to: afreenhashmimgip@gmail.com

IntechOpen

## References

[1] Knopman DS, Petersen RC, Jack CR. A brief history of "Alzheimer disease": Multiple meanings separated by a common name. Neurology. 2019;**92**(22): 1053-1059

[2] Hippius H, Neundörfer G. The discovery of Alzheimer's disease. Dialogues in Clinical Neuroscience. 2003;**5**(1):101-108

[3] Alzheimer's Disease. Mayo Clinic. Mayo Foundation for Medical Education and Research. 2021. Available from: https://www.mayoclinic.org/diseases-conditions/alzheimers-disease/symptoms-causes/syc-20350447 [Accessed: 27 August 2021]

[4] Toepper M. Dissociating normal aging from Alzheimer's disease: A view from cognitive neuroscience. Journal of Alzheimer's Disease. 2017;**57**(2):331-352

[5] Anonymous. Alzheimer's association: Alzheimer's disease facts and figures. Alzheimers Dement. 2020;**16**:391-460

[6] Gairola N, Kothiyal P. Alzheimer's disease: Current perspectives. World Journal of Pharmacy and Pharmaceutical Sciences. 2018;**7**(3):333-349

[7] Piaceri I, Nacmias B, Sorbi S. Genetics of familial and sporadic Alzheimer's disease. Frontiers in Bioscience. 2013;**1**(5): 167-177

[8] Patel HH. Alzheimer disease epidemiology. Available from: https://www.news-medical.net/health/Alzheimers-Disease-Epidemiology.aspx

[9] Edward GA, Gamez N, Escobedo G, Calderon O, Gonzalez IM. Modifiable risk factors for Alzheimer's disease. Frontiers in Aging Neuroscience. 2019;**11**:146

[10] Chen JH, Lin KP, Chen YC. Risk factors for dementia. Journal of the Formosan Medical Association. 2009;**108**(10):754-764

[11] National Institute of Aging. Alzheimer's disease genetic fact sheet. Alzheimer's disease education and referral centre. 2019. Publication No. 11-6424 [Accessed: 12 December 2020]

[12] Wang B. Gene APOE4 causes Alzheimer's disease in humans and a fix has been created. 2018. Available from: https://www.nextbigfuture.com/2018/04/gene-apoe4-causes-alzheimers-disease-in-humans-and-a-fix-has-been-created.html [Accessed: 10 May 2021]

[13] Anonymous. Alzheimer's association: Alzheimer's disease facts and figures. Alzheimers Dement. 2015;**11**:332-384

[14] Nicolas G, Acuña-Hidalgo R, Keogh MJ, Quenez O, Steehouwer M, Lelieveld S, et al. Somatic variants in autosomal dominant genes are a rare cause of sporadic Alzheimer's disease. Alzheimers Dement. 2018;**14**(12): 1632-1639

[15] Menghani YR, Bhattad DM, Chandak KK, Taksande JB, Umekar MJ. A review: Pharmacological and herbal remedies in the management of neurodegenerative disorder (Alzheimer's). International Journal of Pharmacognosy and Life Science. 2021;**2**(1):18-27

[16] https://calgaryguide.ucalgary.ca/alzheimers-disease-pathogenesis-and-clinical-findings/ [Accessed: 21 June 2021]

[17] Imbimbo BP, Lombard J, Pomara N. Pathophysiology of Alzheimer's disease. Neuroimaging Clinics of North America. 2005;**15**(4):727-753

[18] Sajjad R, Arif R, Shah AA, Manzoor I, Mustafa G. Pathogenesis of Alzheimer's disease; Role of amyloid-beta and hyperphosphorylated Tau protein. Indian Journal of Pharmaceutical Sciences. 2018;**80**(4):581-591

[19] Tiwari S, Atluri V, Kaushik A, Yndart A, Nair M. Alzheimer's disease: Pathogenesis, diagnostics and therapeutics. International Journal of Nanomedicine. 2019;**14**:5541-5554

[20] Thakur AK, Kamboj P, Goswami K. Pathophysiology and management of Alzheimer's disease: An overview. Journal of Analytical & Pharmaceutical Research. 2018;**9**(2):226-235

[21] Lipton SA. The molecular basis of memantine action in Alzheimer's disease and other neurologic disorders: Low-affinity, uncompetitive antagonism. Current Alzheimer Research. 2005;**2**:155-165

[22] Santos CY, Snyder PJ, Wu WC, Zhang M, Echeverria A, Alber J. Pathophysiologic relationship between Alzheimer's disease, cerebrovascular disease, and cardiovascular risk: A review and synthesis. Alzheimer's & Dementia: Diagnosis, Assessment & Disease Monitoring. 2017;**7**:69-87

[23] Zhao Y, Zhao B. Oxidative stress and the pathogenesis of Alzheimer's disease. Oxidative Medicine and Cellular Longevity. 2013;**2013**:1-10

[24] Singh RP, Sharad S, Kapur S. Free radicals and oxidative stress in neurodegenerative diseases: Relevance of dietary antioxidants. Journal, Indian Academy of Clinical Medicine. 2004;**5**(3):218-225

[25] Agostinho P, Cunha RA, Oliveria C. Neuroinflammation, oxidative stress and the pathogenesis of Alzheimer's disease. Current Pharmaceutical Design. 2010;**16**(25):2766-2778

[26] Ortiz JMP, Swerdlow RH. Mitochondrial dysfunction in Alzheimer's disease: Role in pathogenesis and novel therapeutic opportunities. British Pharmacological Society. 2019;**176**(18): 3489-3507

[27] Konttinen H, Mauricio CC, Ohtonen S, Wojciechowski S, Shakirzyanova A, Caligola S, et al. PSEN1ΔE9, APPswe, and APOE4 confer disparate phenotypes in human iPSC-derived microglia. Stem Cell Reports. 2019;**13**(4):669-683

[28] Azizi G, Navabi SS, Al-Shukaili A, Seyedzadeh MH, Yazdani R, Mirshafiey A. The role of inflammatory mediators in the pathogenesis of Alzheimer's disease. Sultan Qaboos University Medical Journal. 2015;**15**(3): e305-e316

[29] Akiyama H, Barger S, Barnum S, Bradt B, Bauer J, Cole GM, et al. Inflammation and Alzheimer's disease. Neurobiology of Aging. 2000;**21**(3): 383-421

[30] Perez JMR, Ruiz JMM. A review: Inflammatory process in Alzheimer's disease, role of cytokines. The Scientific World Journal. 2012;**2012**:1-15

[31] Guo L, Zhong MB, Zhang L, Zhang B, Cai D. Sex differences in Alzheimer's disease: Insights from the multiomics landscape. Biological Psychiatry. 2021;**19**(1):61-71

[32] Briggs R, Kennelly SP, O'Neill D. Drug treatments in Alzheimer's disease. Clinical Medicine. 2016;**16**(3):247-253

[33] Lippincott, Williams, and Wilkins. Alzheimer disease drugs. In: Karch AM, editor. Nursing 2010 Drug Handbook. Philadelphia: Wolters Kluwer Health; 2010. pp. 546-551

[34] Jeffrey C, Garam L, Travis M, Aaron R, Kate Z. Alzheimer's disease drug development pipeline: 2017. Alzheimer's & Dementia : Translational Research & Clinical Interventions. 2017;**3**(3):367-384

[35] https://reference.medscape.com/drug/999990 [Accessed: 21 July 2021]

[36] Adlimoghaddam A, Neuendorff M, Roy B, Albensi BC. A review of clinical

treatment considerations of donepezil in severe Alzheimer's disease. CNS Neuroscience & Therapeutics. 2018; **24**(10):876-888

[37] Menting KW, Claassen JAHR. β-secretase inhibitor: A promising novel therapeutic drug in Alzheimer's disease. Frontiers in Aging Neuroscience. 2014;**6**(165):1-9

[38] May PC, Willis BA, Lowe SL, Dean RA, Monk SA, Cocke PJ, et al. The potent BACE1 inhibitor LY2886721 elicits robust central Aβ pharmacodynamics responses in mice, dogs, and humans. The Journal of Neuroscience. 2015;**35**(3):1199-1210

[39] Vassar R, Kandalepas PC. The β-secretase enzyme BACE1 as a therapeutic target for Alzheimer's disease. Alzheimer's Research & Therapy. 2011;**3**(20):1-6

[40] Yan R, Vassar R. Targeting the β secretase BACE1 for Alzheimer's disease therapy. The Lancet Neurology. 2014; **13**(3):319-329

[41] Imbimbo BP, Giardina GAM. γ-secretase inhibitors and modulators for the treatment of Alzheimer's disease: Disappointments and hopes. Current Topics in Medicinal Chemistry. 2011;**11**(12):1555-1570

[42] Wolfe MS. γ-secretase as a target for Alzheimer's disease. Advances in Pharmacology. 2012;**64**(127):127-153

[43] Doody RS, Raman R, Farlow M, Iwatsubo T, Vellas B, Joffe S, et al. A phase 3 trial of semagacestat for treatment of Alzheimer's disease. The New England Journal of Medicine. 2013;**369**(4):341-350

[44] Coric V, Dyck CHV, Salloway S, Andreasen N, Brody M, Richter RW, et al. Safety and tolerability of the γ-secretase inhibitor avagacestat in a phase 2 study of mild to moderate

Alzheimer disease. Archives of Neurology. 2012;**69**(11):1430-1440

[45] Dockens R, Wang JS, Castaneda L, Sverdlov O, Huang SP, Slemmon R, et al. A placebo-controlled, multiple ascending dose study to evaluate the safety, pharmacokinetics and pharmacodynamics of avagacestat (BMS-708163) in healthy young and elderly subjects. Clinical Pharmaco-kinetics. 2012;**51**(10):681-693

[46] Tong G, Castaneda L, Wang JS, Sverdlov O, Huang SP, Slemmon R, et al. Effects of single doses of avagacestat (BMS-708163) on cerebrospinal fluid Aβ levels in healthy young men. Clinical Drug Investigation. 2012;**32**(11):761-769

[47] Jaturapatporn D, Isaac MGEKN, McCleery J, Tabet N. Aspirin, steroidal and non-steroidal anti-inflammatory drugs for the treatment of Alzheimer's disease. Cochrane Database of Systematic Reviews. 2012;**2**:CD006378

[48] Miguel-´Alvarez M, Santos-Lozano A, Sanchis-Gomar F, Fiuza-Luces C, Pareja-Galeano H, Garatachea N, et al. Non-steroidal anti-inflammatory drugs as a treatment for Alzheimer's disease: A systematic review and meta-analysis of treatment effect. Drugs & Aging. 2015;**32**(2): 139-147

[49] Pasqualetti P, Bonomini C, Forno GD, Paulon L, Sinforiani E, Marra C, et al. A randomized controlled study on effects of ibuprofen on cognitive progression of Alzheimer's disease. Aging Clinical and Experimental Research. 2009;**21**(2):102-110

[50] Matlack KES, Tardiff DF, Narayan P, Hamamichi S, Caldwell KA, Lindquist S. Clioquinol promotes the degradation of metal-dependent amyloid-β (Aβ) oligomers to restore endocytosis and ameliorate Aβ toxicity. Proceedings of the National Academy of Sciences of the United States of America. 2014;**111**(11): 4013-4018

[51] Robert A, Liu Y, Nguyen M, Meunier B. Regulation of copper and iron homeostasis by metal chelators: A possible chemotherapy for Alzheimer's disease. Accounts of Chemical Research. 2015;**48**(5):1332-1339

[52] Ryan TM, Roberts BR, McColl G, Hare DJ, Doble PA, Li QX, et al. Stabilization of nontoxic Aβ-oligomers: Insights into the mechanism of action of hydroxyquinolines in Alzheimer's disease. The Journal of Neuroscience. 2015;**35**(7):2871-2884

[53] Galasko D, Bell J, Mancuso JY, Kupiec JW, Sabbagh MN, Dyck CV, et al. Clinical trial of an inhibitor of RAGE-Aβ interactions in Alzheimer disease. Neurology. 2014;**82**(17):1536-1542

[54] Dearie R, Sagare A, Zlokovic BV. The role of the cell surface LRP and soluble LRP in blood-brain barrier Aβ clearance in Alzheimer's disease. Current Pharmaceutical Design. 2008;**14**(16): 1601-1605

[55] Gilman S, Koller M, Black RS, Jenkins L, Griffith SG, Fox NC, et al. Clinical effects of Aβ immunization (AN1792) in patients with AD in an interrupted trial. Neurology. 2005;**64**(9):1553-1562

[56] Wiessner C, Wiederhold KH, Tissot AC, Frey P, Danner S, Jacobson LH, et al. The second generation active Aβ immunotherapy CAD106 reduces amyloid accumulation in APP transgenic mice while minimizing potential side effects. Journal of Neuroscience. 2011;**31**(25):9323-9331

[57] Panza F, Solfrizzi V, Imbimbo BP, Logroscino G. Amyloid-directed monoclonal antibodies for the treatment of Alzheimer's disease: The point of no return? Expert Opinion on Biological Therapy. 2014;**14**(10):1465-1476

[58] Panza F, Solfrizzi V, Imbimbo BP, Tortelli R, Santamato A, Logroscino G.

Amyloid-based immunotherapy for Alzheimer's disease in the time of prevention trials: The way forward. Expert Review of Clinical Immunology. 2014;**10**(3):405-419

[59] Salloway S, Sperling R, Fox NC, et al. Two phase 3 trials of bapineuzumab in mild-to-moderate Alzheimer's disease. The New England Journal of Medicine. 2014;**370**(4):322-333

[60] Doody RS, Thomas RG, Farlow M, Iwatsubo T, Vellas B, Joffe S, et al. Phase 3 trials of solanezumab for mild-to-moderate Alzheimer's disease. The New England Journal of Medicine. 2014;**370**(4):311-321

[61] Tayeb HO, Murray ED, Price BH, Tarazi FI. Bapineuzumab and solanezumab for Alzheimer's disease: Is the 'amyloid cascade hypothesis' still alive? Expert Opinion on Biological Therapy. 2013;**13**(7):1075-1084

[62] Jindal H, Bhatt B, Malik JS. Alzheimer disease immunotherapeutics: Then and now. Human Vaccines & Immuno-therapeutics. 2014;**10**(9):2741-2743

[63] Cowan CM, Mudher A. Are tau aggregates toxic or protective in tauopathies? Frontiers in Neurology. 2013;**4**(114):1-13

[64] West S, Bhugra P. Emerging drug targets for Aβ and tau in Alzheimer's disease: A systematic review. British Journal of Clinical Pharmacology. 2015;**80**(2):221-234

[65] Shefet-Carasso L, Benhar I. Antibody-targeted drugs and drug resistance-challenges and solutions. Drug Resistance Updates. 2015;**18**:36-46

[66] Mehta DC, Short JL, Hilmer SN, Nicolazzo JA. Drug access to the central nervous system in Alzheimer's disease: Preclinical and clinical insights. Pharmaceutical Research. 2015;**32**(3): 819-839

[67] Berk C, Paul G, Sabbagh M. Investigational drugs in Alzheimer's disease: Current progress. Expert Opinion on Investigational Drugs. 2014;**23**(6):837-846

[68] Grüninger F. Invited review: Drug development for tauopathies. Neuropathology and Applied Neurobiology. 2015;**41**(1):81-96

[69] Iqbal K, Gong CX, Liu F. Microtubule-associated protein tau as a therapeutic target in Alzheimer's disease. Expert Opinion on Therapeutic Targets. 2014;**18**(3):307-318

[70] Kimura T, Ishiguro K, Hisanaga SI. Physiological and pathological phosphorylation of tau by Cdk5. Frontiers in Molecular Neuroscience. 2014;**7**(65):1-10

[71] Resnick L, Fennell M. Targeting JNK3 for the treatment of neurodegenerative disorders. Drug Discovery Today. 2004;**9**(21):932-939

[72] Baddeley TC, McCaffrey J, Storey JMD, Cheung JKS, Melis V, Horsley D, et al. Complex disposition of methylthioninium redox forms determines efficacy in tau aggregation inhibitor therapy for Alzheimer's disease. The Journal of Pharmacology and Experimental Therapeutics. 2015;**352**(1):110-118

[73] Wischik CM, Staff RT, Wischik DJ, Bentham P, Murray AD, Storey JMD, et al. Tau aggregation inhibitor therapy: An exploratory phase 2 study in mild or moderate Alzheimer's disease. Journal of Alzheimer's Disease. 2015;**44**(2):705-720

[74] Shemesh OA, Spira ME. Rescue of neurons from undergoing hallmark tau-induced Alzheimer's disease cell pathologies by the antimitotic drug paclitaxel. Neurobiology of Disease. 2011;**43**(1):163-175

[75] Wisniewski T, Goni F. Immunotherapeutic approaches for Alzheimer's disease. Neuron. 2015; **85**(6):1162-1176

[76] Kontsekova E, Zilka N, Kovacech B, Novak P, Novak M. First-in-man tau vaccine targeting structural determinants essential for pathological tau-tau interaction reduces tau oligomerisation and neurofibrillary degeneration in an Alzheimer's disease model. Alzheimer's Research & Therapy. 2014;**6**(4):44

[77] Tata AM, Velluto L, D'angelo C, Reale M. Cholinergic system dysfunction and neurodegenerative diseases: Cause or effect? CNS & Neurological Disorders Drug Targets. 2014;**13**(7):1294-1303

[78] Wallace TL, Bertrand D. Importance of the nicotinic acetylcholine receptor system in the prefrontal cortex. Biochemical Pharmacology. 2013; **85**(12):1713-1720

[79] Lourenco MV, Ferreira ST, DeFelice FG. Neuronal stress signaling and eIF2$\alpha$ phosphorylation as molecular links between Alzheimer's disease and diabetes. Progress in Neurobiology. 2015;**129**:37-57

[80] Hokama M, Oka S, Leon J. Altered expression of diabetes-related genes in Alzheimer's disease brains: The Hisayama study. Cerebral Cortex. 2014;**24**(9):2476-2488

[81] Lourenco MV, Clarke JR, Frozza RL, Bomfim TR, Forny-Germano L, Batista AF, et al. TNF-$\alpha$ mediates PKR-dependent memory impairment and brain IRS-1 inhibition induced by Alzheimer's $\beta$-amyloid oligomers in mice and monkeys. Cell Metabolism. 2013;**18**(6):831-843

[82] Gold M, Alderton C, Zvartau-Hind M, Egginton S, Saunders AM, Irizarry M, et al. Rosiglitazone monotherapy in mild-to-moderate Alzheimer's disease: Results from a randomized, double-blind,

placebo-controlled phase III study. Dementia and Geriatric Cognitive Disorders. 2010;**30**(2):131-146

[83] Blalock EM, Phelps JT, Pancani T, Searcy JL, Anderson KL, Gant JC, et al. Effects of longterm pioglitazone treatment on peripheral and central markers of aging. PLoS One. 2010;**5**(4): e10405

[84] Qin W, Haroutunian V, Katsel P, Cardozo CP, Ho L, Buxbaum JD, et al. PGC-1α expression decreases in the Alzheimer disease brain as a function of dementia. Archives of Neurology. 2009;**66**(3):352-361

[85] Katsouri L, Parr C, Bogdanovic N, Willem M, Sastre M. PPARγ co-activator-1α (PGC-1α) reduces amyloid-β generation through a PPARγ-dependent mechanism. Journal of Alzheimer's Disease. 2011;**25**(1):151-162

[86] Sato T, Hanyu H, Hirao K, Kanetaka H, Sakurai H, Iwamoto T. Efficacy of PPAR-γ agonist pioglitazone in mild Alzheimer disease. Neurobiology of Aging. 2011;**32**(9):1626-1633

[87] Claxton A, Baker LD, Hanson A, Trittschuh EH, Cholerton B, Morgan A, et al. Long-acting intranasal insulin detemir improves cognition for adults with mild cognitive impairment or early-stage Alzheimer's disease dementia. Journal of Alzheimer's Disease. 2015;**44**(3):897-906

[88] Qiu WQ, Zhu H. Amylin and its analogs: A friend or foe for the treatment of Alzheimer's disease? Frontiers in Aging Neuroscience. 2014;**6**:186

[89] Valu M, Ducu C, Moga S, Negree D, Hritcu L, Boiangiu RS, et al. Effects of the hydroethanolic extract of *Lycopodium selago* L. on scopolamine-induced memory deficits in Zebrafish. Multidisciplinary Digital Publishing Institute. 2021;**14**(6):1-22

[90] Datta S, Patil S. Evaluation of traditional herb extract *Salvia officinalis* in treatment of Alzheimer's disease. Pharmacognosy Journal. 2020;**12**(1): 131-143

[91] Wang L, Jin GF, Yu HH, Lu XH, Zou ZH, Liang JQ, et al. Protective effects of tenuifolin isolated from *Polygala tenuifolia* Willd roots on neuronal apoptosis and learning and memory deficits in mice with Alzheimer's disease. Food & Function. 2019;**10**(11):7453-7460

[92] Kizhakke AP, Olakkaran S, Antony A, Tilagul S, Hunasanahally G. *Convolvulus pluricaulis* (Shankhapushpi) ameliorates human microtubule-associated protein tau (hMAPτ) induced neurotoxicity in Alzheimer's disease Drosophila model. Journal of Chemistry Neuroanatomy. 2019;**95**:115-122

[93] Medrano-Jiménez E, Carrillo IJF, Pedraza-Escalona M, Ramírez-Serrano CE, Álvarez-Arellano L, Cortés-Mendoza J, et al. *Malva parviflora* extract ameliorates the deleterious effects of a high fat diet on the cognitive deficit in a mouse model of Alzheimer's disease by restoring microglial function via a PPAR-γ-dependent mechanism. Journal of Neuroinflammation. 2019;**16**(143):1-26

[94] Pal G, Pradeep AK. Antioxidant, anti-Alzheimer and anti-Parkinson of *Artemisia nilagirica* leaves with flowering tops. UK Journal of Pharmaceutical and Biosciences. 2018;**6**(2):12-23

[95] Akinyemi AJ, Faboya L, Awonegan AP, Olayide I. Antioxidant and anti-acetylcholinesterase activities of essential oils from garlic (*Allium sativum*) bulbs. International Journal of Plant Research. 2018;**31**(2):1-10

[96] Parameshwari K, Kumar S, Priyadharshini Bai G, Prathima C, Neetha C. Nootropic activity of ethanolic extract of *Alangium*

*salvifolium* leaves on Scopolamine mouse model of Alzheimer's disease. National Journal of Physiology, Pharmacy and Pharmacology. 2018;**8**(12):1625-1630

[97] Mahaman YAR, Huang F, Wu M, Wang Y, Wei Z, Bao J, et al. *Moringa oleifera* alleviates homocysteine-induced Alzheimer's disease-like pathology and cognitive impairment. Journal of Alzheimer's Disease. 2018;**63**(3):1141-1159

[98] Manasa A, Karimulla SK, Gobinath M. Ameliorative effect of *Cleome gynandra* Linn against scopolamine induced amnesia in mice. International Journal of Research in Pharmacy and Science. 2017;**8**(4):642-649

[99] Kaura S, Parle M. Evaluation of nootropic potential of green peas in mice. Journal of Applied Pharmaceutical Science. 2017;**7**(5):166-173

[100] Phetcharat B, Wanida S, Supita T, Pennapa C. Ameliorative effect of *Apium graveolens* Linn on scopolamine-induced amnesia mice. International Conference on Herbal and Traditional Medicine. 2017;**10**(10):82-93

[101] Jyothi CH, Shashikala G, Vidya HK, Shashikala GH. Evaluation of effect of alcoholic extract of *Tinospora cordifolia* on learning and memory in alprazolam induced amnesia in albino mice. International Journal of Basic & Clinical Pharmacology. 2016;**5**(5):2159-2163

[102] Mahmoodzadeh T, Kashani MHK, Ramshini H, Moslem A, Zadeh MM. Effect of *Camellia sinensis* on spatial memory in a rat model of Alzheimer's disease. Journal of Biomedical Science. 2016;**1**(1):e5340

[103] Reddy N, Sultanpur CM, Saritha V. Evaluation of nootropic activity of *Curcuma longa* leaves in diazepam and scopolamine-induced amnesic mice and rats. International Journal of Basic & Clinical Pharmacology. 2015;**4**(4):714-719

[104] Nemalapalli Y, Shaik A, Kadrivel D, Kumar D, Sundararajan P, Balagani PK. Effect of ethanolic seed extract of *Bauhinia purpurea* Linn on cognition in scopolamine induced Alzheimer's disease rat's model. Journal of Comprehensive Pharmacy. 2015;**2**(4):145-150

[105] Kim HG, Park G, Lim S, Park H, Choi JG, UkJeong H, et al. *Mori fructus* improves cognitive and neuronal dysfunction induced by beta-amyloid toxicity through the GSK-3β pathway in vitro and in vivo. Journal of Ethnopharmacology. 2015;**171**:196-204

[106] Oboh G, Ayodele J, Akinyemi OS, Oyeleye S. Anticholinesterase and antioxidative properties of aqueous extract of *Cola acuminata* seed *in vitro*. International Journal of Alzheimer's Disease. 2014:498629

[107] Ramachandran S, Sanjay S, Dhanaraju M. Antiamnesic effect of piracetam potentiated with *Emblica officinalis* and *Curcuma longa* in aluminium induced neurotoxicity of Alzheimer's disease. International Journal of Advanced Research. 2013;**1**(7):185-196

[108] Alikatte KL, Akondi BR, Yerragunta VG, Veerareddy PR, Palle S. Antiamnesic activity of *Syzygium cumini* against scopolamine induced spatial memory impairments in rats. Brain & Development. 2012;**34**(10):844-851

[109] Faiyaz A, Narendra J, Sharath C. Acetylcholine and memory-enhancing activity of *Ficus racemosa* bark. Pharmacognosy Research. 2011;**3**(4): 246-249

[110] Muralidharan P, Kumar VR, Balamurugan G. Protective effect of *Morinda citrifolia* fruits on β-amyloid (25-35) induced cognitive dysfunction in mice: An experimental and biochemical study. Phytotherapy Research. 2010;**24**(2):252-258

[111] https://dailymed.nlm.nih.gov/dailymed/drugInfo.cfm?

setid=41706573-546f-6774-6872-5374726f6e67 [Accessed: 18 January 2022]

[112] Alzheimer's Association. Aducanumab approved for treatment of Alzheimer's disease. Available from: https://www.alz.org/alzheimers-dementia/treatments/aducanumab [Accessed: 10 September 2021]

[113] https://jamanetwork.com/journals/jamaneurology/fullarticle/2783263 [Accessed: 10 September 2021]

[114] Huang LK, Chao SP, Hu CJ. Clinical trials of new drugs for Alzheimer disease. Journal of Biomedical Science. 2020;**27**(18):1-13

[115] Cumming J, Lee G, Zhong K, Fonseca J, Taghva K. Alzheimer's disease drug development pipeline: 2021. Alzheimer's & Dementia. 2021;7:e12179

Chapter 4

# MicroRNAs as Future Treatment Tools and Diagnostic Biomarkers in Alzheimer's Disease

*Heena Chauhan, Pawan Gupta and Bhagawati Saxena*

## Abstract

Alzheimer's disease (AD) is a neurodegenerative disorder and is considered to be the most common form of dementia. This disorder is characterized by the formation of amyloid β (Aβ) plaques, neurofibrillary tangles, and alterations in synaptic function, all of which cause memory loss and behavioral disturbances. Despite the high prevalence of AD, effective therapeutic and diagnostic tools remain unavailable. MicroRNAs (miRNAs, miRs) are regulatory non-coding RNAs that target mRNAs. MiRNAs are involved in the regulation of the expressions of APP and BACE1, Aβ clearance, and the formation of neuro-fibrillary tangles. Furthermore, there are evidences that show alteration in the expression of several miRs in AD. MicroRNA is emerging as a biomarker because they have high specificity and, efficiency, and can be detected in biological fluids such as cerebrospinal fluid, tear, urine, blood. Moreover, miRNAs may be acquired and measured easily by utilizing real-time PCR, next-generation sequencing, or microarray. These techniques are cost-effective in comparison with imaging techniques such as magnetic resonance imaging, positron emission tomography. These features make miRNAs viable therapeutic as well as diagnostic tools in the treatment of AD. This review covers the regulatory function of miRNAs in AD, as well as their prospective applications as diagnostic biomarkers.

**Keywords:** Alzheimer's disease, dementia, pathogenesis, microRNAs, diagnosis, biomarker

## 1. Introduction

Alzheimer's disease (AD) is a neurodegenerative disorder and is considered to be the most common form of dementia that majorly occurs in aged persons although a familial form of AD can occur in the younger population. Familial (early-onset) AD occurs due to mutations in the amyloid precursor protein (APP), presenilin 1, and presenilin 2 genes [1]. However, further identification of tau gene mutations in familial frontotemporal dementia (FTD) with chromosome 17 has shown a clear relationship between tau malfunction and dementia [2]. These findings show that AD and FTD are related in a hereditary spectrum of degenerative brain illnesses in which tau appears to play a key role [3]. Clinical manifestations of AD include a slow and persistent deterioration in memory, executive functions, and the capacity to carry out daily activities [4, 5]. Dementia affects around 36.5 million individuals worldwide in 2010. Every 20 years, the number of dementia cases is expected to roughly quadruple, reaching 65.7 million in 2030 and 115.4 million in 2050. AD is accounting for the preponderance of these dementia instances, accounting for 60–80% of all dementia cases [6]. Every year, an estimated 5–7 million new instances of AD are diagnosed in the elderly population [7]. In 2020, overall healthcare expenditures for AD treatment are predicted to be $305 billion, with expenditure expected to rise to more than $1 trillion as the population ages [8]. Even moderate developments in preventative and therapeutic techniques that postpone the initiation and advancement of AD can considerably lower the illness's worldwide impact [9].

## 2. Pathophysiology involved in AD

The scientific field dedicated for understanding the mechanisms involved in the progression of AD and developing relevant therapeutics is vast. Pathologically hallmarks of AD include the extra-neuronal clustering of Aβ plaques and the formation of intraneuronal neurofibrillary tangles (NFTs) which result in neuronal synaptic dysfunction [10, 11]. Aβ plaques formation is found in basal ganglia, amygdala, diencephalon, hippocampus, temporal and later it is found in the brain stem, cerebellar cortex and mesencephalon. The high levels of Aβ plaques are responsible for tau formation in the entorhinal, transentorhinal as well as locus coeruleus areas of the brain. It spreads to the hippocampus and neocortex in the critical stage [12].

Aβ plaque is formed from proteolysis of APP followed by two pathways (1) non-amyloidogenic pathway (physiological pathway), (2) amyloidogenic pathway (**Figure 1**). APP is a transmembrane glycoprotein whose a large portion toward the cytoplasm and a short portion inside the lumen. The non-amyloidogenic pathway prevents to the formation of toxic Aβ as APP is first cleaved by α-secretase and generates soluble fragments sAPPα and C83. These further cleaved by γ-secretase and produced non-toxic p3 and APP Intracellular Domain (AICD). On the other hand, the amyloidogenic pathway, neurotoxic Aβ formed through cleavage of APP by β-secretase (BACE1) followed by γ-secretase and formed sAPPβ, C99, Aβ, and AICD. These fragments are functionally active and influence or modulate signaling proteins [13]. Aβ oligomerization led to the formation of senile plaques and blockage the nerve transmission. There are mainly two types of Aβ isoforms soluble Aβ40 and insoluble Aβ42. The latter Aβ is more prone to aggregate and high concentration found in AD patients [14, 15]. The Aβ polymers aggregation results in blockage of ion channel, decreased energy metabolism, alteration in calcium homeostasis, diminish glucose regulation, and increases mitochondrial stress level, which further plays role in abnormality in neuronal health and causes neuronal death [12, 16]. Moreover, the AICD acts differently according to its generating pathways. The AICD from non-amyloidogenic pathways is degrading rapidly, but in the case of the amyloidogenic pathway, AICD behaves as a regulator for other genes [17].

Intra-neuronal deposition of NFTs are another pathophysiological hallmark of AD. NFTs were predominantly consisted of hyper-phosphorylated tau due to imbalance between phosphorylation and de-phosphorylation of tau [18]. Kinases are involved in the phosphorylation of tau protein, while phosphatases remove the phosphate residues. Tau proteins are microtubule-associated proteins that help vesicle transportation by stabilizing the microtubule. Microtubules are essential for axonal transport, neuronal structure, and neural plasticity [19]. Heavily phosphorylated tau may lose its capacity to stabilize itself and begin to self-form NFTs. Neurons cannot operate correctly without a full system of microtubules, and they eventually die. Tauopathies are considered to be an indicator of the severity of AD [20].

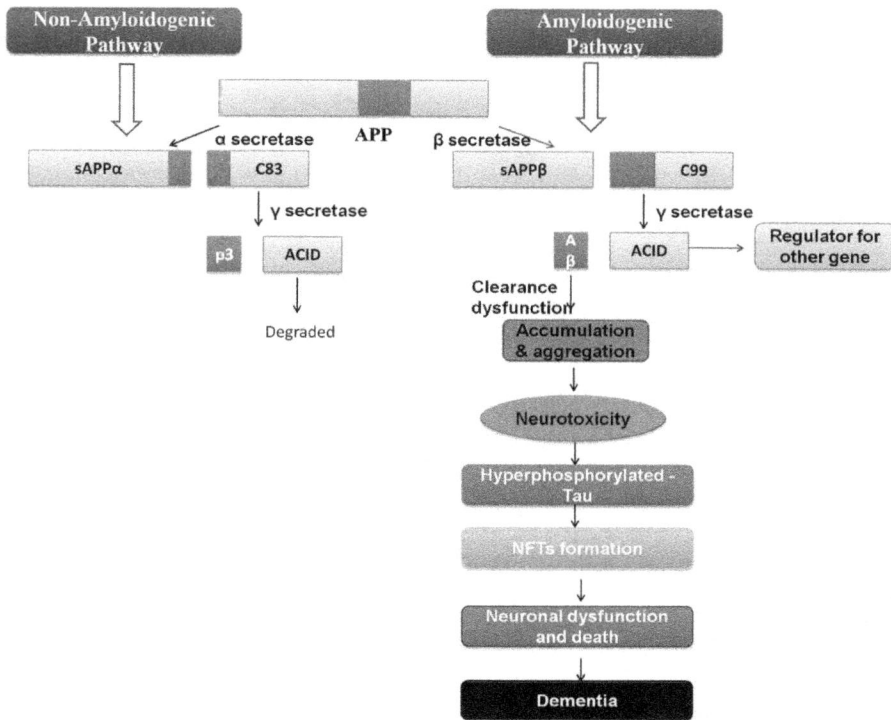

**Figure 1.**
*Amyloidogenic and non-amyloidogenic pathways. APP = amyloid precursor protein; ACID = APP intracellular domain; NFTs = neurofibrillary tangles.*

## 3. MicroRNA

MicroRNA (miRNA/miR) is a kind of non-coding RNA that has 22–23 nucleotides. They regulate gene expression by interacting with the 3′-untranslated region (3′UTR) of mRNA. Thus, miRNA inhibits translation or destroys the targeted mRNA as a result of this event [21, 22]. Biogenesis of miRNA occurs with both canonical pathways as well as non-canonical pathways. However, miRNAs are processed dominantly by the canonical biogenesis pathway [23]. The detailed process of miRNA biogenesis by canonical pathway is illustrated in **Figure 2**. RNA polymerase II in the nucleus transcribed miRNAs gene to primary miRNAs (pri-miRNAs). In collaboration with Pasha/DGCR8, the RNase III enzyme, Drosha converts these pri-miRNAs into precursor miRNAs (pre-miRNAs) and then these pre-miRNAs are transported to the cytoplasm by Exportin 5 [24, 25]. These pre-miRNAs are of approximately 70 nucleotides in a hairpin structure. Pre-miRNAs features a hairpin loop structure that is identified by dicer present in the cytoplasm for cleavage, resulting in the formation of mature miRNAs which is a double-stranded miRNA duplex [25]. The miRNA-induced silencing complex (miRISC) is formed when one of these strands of the mature duplex is loaded onto a member of the Argonaute (Ago) family of proteins, whereas the other strand of the mature duplex is normally destroyed. RISCs mediate gene silencing by recognizing the 3′ untranslated region (3′ UTR) of target mRNA [24, 25].

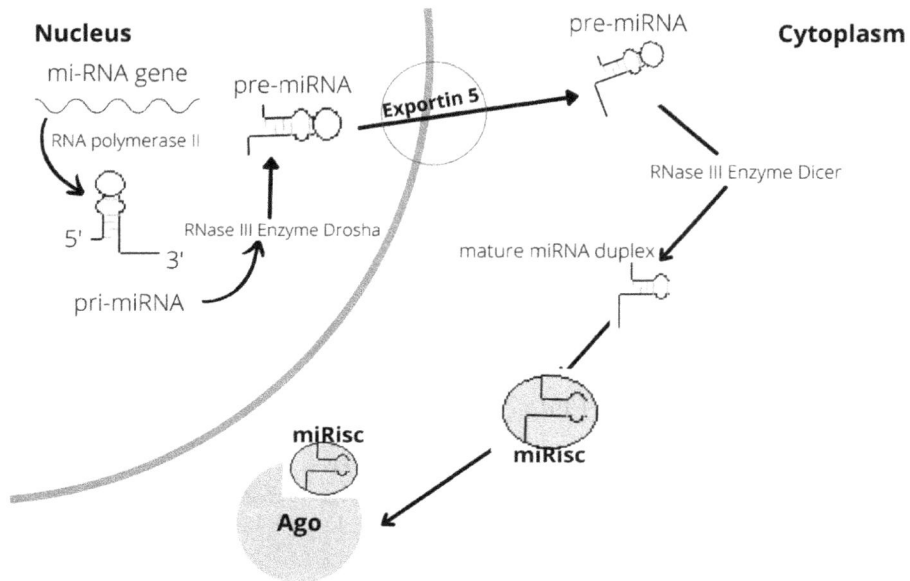

**Figure 2.**
*Schematic diagram of miRNA synthesis; ago: argonaute protein; miRisc: RNA-induced silencing complex.*

## 4. Association of microRNAs and Alzheimer's disease

Pathologically, AD is generated by impaired metabolism of Aβ and the imbalance between the hyper-phosphorylated and de-phosphorylated forms of tau. Although these clinical-pathological features of AD are extensively established, therapies aiming at lowering synthesis or eliminating misfolded proteins are very limited [21]. Only four medicines, including three cholinesterase inhibitors (donepezil, rivastigmine, and galanthamine) and the glutamate regulator memantine, were licensed by the US Food and Drug Administration (FDA) for the treatment of cognitive impairment and dysfunction in symptomatic AD until June 2021. These symptomatic therapies can only delay rather than stop disease development [26, 27]. On June 7, 2021, Aducanumab, the first targeted Alzheimer's therapy was approved by the FDA to treat patients with AD [27]. Thus, a different approach has centred on genetics, with several genes encoding proteins in central nervous system (CNS ) offered as candidates to explain AD etiology [21]. Earlier studies showed miRNA play role in the elaborating different types of pathogenic diseases including cardiovascular, cancer, and neurological disorders [28, 29]. Numbers of studies show the involvement of miRNAs in the pathogenesis and their therapeutic potential in various neurodegenerative diseases including AD, Huntington's disease, Parkinson's disease, amyotrophic lateral sclerosis, and Prion diseases [30, 31]. AD study indicates that miRNA may be helpful for the regulation of genes, expressions of proteins, and changes in phenotype in human diseases. Some research studies show the abnormal regulation of miRNA-dependent genes which are responsible for the formation and deposition of Aβ plaques as well as NFTs and consequently neuronal-degeneration [32–35]. The focus of this review is the implication of the miRNAs in the two most well-recognized theories of AD pathogenesis: the Aβ hypothesis (**Figure 3**) and the tau hypothesis (**Figure 4**).

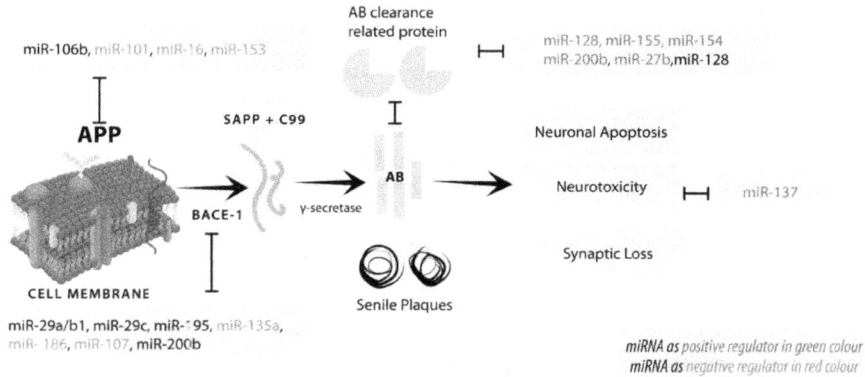

**Figure 3.**
*A schematic diagram of the Aβ hypothesis in AD pathogenesis and involvement of miRNA in each stage. The amyloid beta is produced as a result of processing the APP (amyloid precursor protein) by a sequential enzyme digested by BACE1 and γ-secretase generate imbalance between the clearance and production of Aβ which is the key factor of AD.*

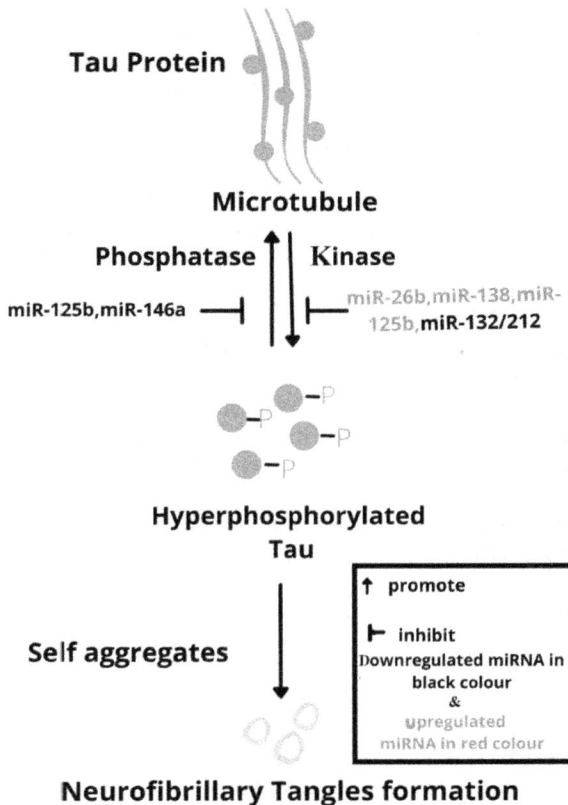

**Figure 4.**
*The imbalance between the hyper-phosphorylated and de-phosphorylated processes of Tau could lead to the formation of NFTs. The miRNAs involved in the phosphorylated and de-phosphorylated processes play a role in AD pathogenesis.*

## 4.1 MicroRNAs involved in the regulation of APP expression

Although APP regulation is challenging, the research of regulatory processes indicate the prognosis of Alzheimer's patients (**Figure 3**). Some scientific evidence shows that miR-106b regulates APP expression by binding on the 3′UTR region of APP [33]. The miR-101 [36], miR-16 [37], and miR-153 [38] are found APP negative regulators in in-vitro studies as well as in-vivo studies.

## 4.2 MicroRNAs involved in the regulation of BACE1 expression

It has been found that BACE-1 expression and activity are regulated by some miRNAs like the miR-29 family. BACE-1 expression level is increased with decreased expression of miR29a/b1 in sporadic AD brain. Moreover, it was also validated that low-level expression of miR29a/b1 is responsible for the pathogenesis of AD by promoting the production of Aβ plaques [39]. Another study found that downregulation of BACE1 is found in a cell line (SH-SY5Y) with overexpression of miR-29c via binding of BACE-13′ UTR [40]. Another study revealed that miR-107 regulates the expression of BACE1 in cell culture by binding the 3′UTR of BACE1 [41]. It was demonstrated that the BACE1 mRNA level was negatively affected by miR-107. Therefore, miR-107 could be a potential drug target [42] as it prevents the Aβ induced neurotoxicity and blood barrier dysfunction [43]. Certain miRNAs which are negative regulators of BACE1 expression by binding with 3′ UTR of BACE1 include miR-298/328 [44], miR-135a [45], miR135b [46], miR-186 [47], miR-195 [48], miR-200b [45], and miR-339-5P (**Figure 3**) [49].

## 4.3 Role of MicroRNAs in Aβ clearance

The deposition of Aβ occurred due to an imbalance between production and clearance of Aβ. Several studies show that certain microRNAs are involved in the clearance of Aβ. The upregulation of miR-128 can alter the Aβ clearance by targeting the lysosomal enzyme system in monocytes of AD sporadic patients. The breakdown of Aβ plaque in Alzheimer's patients improves when miR-128 is blocked in monocytes [50]. In addition, miR-34a was also involved in digesting the Aβ, thus improving the clearance of overexpressed Aβ [51]. miR-155, 154, 200b, 27b, 128 immune-related microRNA allegedly contribute to the process of Aβ clearance mediated by blood-derived monocytes (BDMs) when expressed variably in the CCL2/CCR2 (chemokine/chemokine receptor) axis [52]. miR-302 may attenuate Aβ induced neuronal toxicity in the brain of Alzheimer's patients via PTEN/ AKT/ Nrf2/Ho-1 pathway. miR-137 may reduced Aβ induced toxicity of neurons with the help of NF-kβ by TNFAIP1 expression repressing in N2a cells [53].

## 4.4 MicroRNAs targeting neurofibrillary tangles

The expression levels of miR 26b [54], miR-125b [55, 56], miR-138 [57], and miR-146a [58] have been shown to be considerably up-regulated while miR-132/212 down-regulated [59] in Alzheimer's patients. Overexpression of miR-125b inhibited the two phosphatases i.e., PPP1CA and DUSP6 which further causes tau hyperphosphorylation while kinase expression/activity and tau phosphorylation were reduced when miR-125b was inhibited [55]. miR-146a was discovered to specifically target the coiled-coil containing protein kinase1 (ROCK1) in brain cells, and inhibiting ROCK1 might cause aberrant tau phosphorylation [58]. Reports showed that miR-138 was found to promote tau phosphorylation via directly targeting the retinoic acid receptor alpha (RARA)/ glycogen synthase kinase-3b (GSK-3b) pathway in HEK293/tau and N2a/APP cells [57].

The increased levels of miR-26b in post-mitotic neurons led to the pathophysiology of AD via cell cycle entrance, tau hyper-phosphorylation, and death [54] (**Figure 4**).

## 5. MicroRNAs as possible treatment tools in Alzheimer's disease

The usage of miRNA in the treatment of the disorder is developing fast. In 2018, the FDA accepted the primary miRNA-founded therapy for the cure of the infrequent progressive polyneuropathy produced by hereditary transthyretin-mediated amyloidosis (hATTR) known as amyloid polyneuropathy [60]. The fact that miRNAs alter (or control) the expression of potential genes in AD has prompted researchers to pursue miRNA-based therapeutic options. The treatment modifications of miRNA are carried out in two different ways: first, the functioning of miRNAs is suppressed by oligonucleotides that target miRNAs are known as antagomirs while in a second way, synthetic oligonucleotides are used which plays the same role as endogenous miRNA (act as miRNA mimics) [61, 62]. Thus, a miRNA mimetic or antagonist could be evaluated as a treatment tool. It was also observed that increased miRNA expression can counter the accumulation of Aβ and tau in cell and animal models of AD. In transgenic mice model, the family of miR-200 (miR-200b and miR-200c) were recognized as Aβ secretion regulators by modulating mTOR in primary type of neurons [63–65]. The same effect of down-regulation in Aβ production was seen after miR-330 upregulation in mice model of AD by activating the MAPK pathway [66]. In in-vitro AD model, inhibition of Aβ accumulation was observed by miR-15b by targeting enzyme BACE1 and NF-κB signaling [67]. Similarly, in-vitro studies suggested that miR-124 works as a basic regulating factor in process of AD by targeting BACE1 and controlling BACE1 gene expression [68]. To understand the contribution of miR-124 in the pathogenesis of AD, the brain tissues of 35 cases of sporadic AD and control subjects were analyzed for miR-124 expression by the qRT-PCR technique. The reduction in the level of miR-124 expression was seen in AD brain tissues with comparison to the control group. In addition, inhibition of miR-124 significantly increased BACE1 levels in human neuroblastoma cells (SH-SY5Y), while miR-124 overexpression significantly suppressed BACE1 [69]. MiR-219 was shown to be downregulated in severe primary age-related tau pathology as evaluated by the RT-qPCR study. In addition, it was shown in the Drosophila model (which produces human tau) that the reduction of miR-219 increases tau toxicity, while the overexpression of miR-219 partially reverses this effect [70]. In in-vivo studies for cognitive capacity in SAMP8 mice, it was found that the miR-214-3p suppresses the autophagy and apoptosis of hippo-campus neurons in sporadic Alzheimer's disease (SAD) [71]. It was also found that miR-let-7f-5p had anti-apoptotic and protective effect in Aβ induced neurotoxicity on grafted mesenchymal stem cells by targeting caspase-3 in AD model [72]. These findings suggested that miR-214-3p and let-7f-5p are having anti-apoptotic activity and increase the cell viability of neurons, therefore, it can be therapeutically important [71, 72]. One literature reported that NF-kB was inactivated by upregulation of PPAR-γ in mouse cortical neurons and Neuro2a cells. MiR-128 targeted the PPAR-γ and by targeting PPAR-gamma reduced the Aβ mediated cytotoxicity in the studies [73]. It was observed that overexpression of both miR-125b [55] and miR-146a [58] stimulates the apoptosis of neuron and tau phosphorylation in cellular and molecular AD models. In recent years many chemicals are studied that can affect miRNAs pharmacologically. Anti-inflammatory medications may be effective in preventing the course of AD through modulating miRNAs. Additionally, naturally obtained compounds are recognized for their possible effect as neuroprotective agents in AD, like resveratrol [74] and osthole [75], which appear to be effective by modulating a specific type of miRNA and activate processes like autophagy and neuronal regeneration. Exosomes, tiny vesicles generated by neurons and glial cells, may also be used as therapies to give miRNAs and/or short interfering RNA (siRNA) to patients, according to new research. Multitargeted treatment methods, such as the use of acetylcholinesterase (AChE) inhibitors in conjunction with the manipulation of certain miRNAs, are also being investigated. Approaching miRNAs as therapeutic targets has two major drawbacks: (1) their ability to control several transcripts (up to hundreds) at once, and (2) the difficulty of achieving effective miRNA delivery.

## 6. MicroRNAs as possible diagnostic biomarkers in Alzheimer's disease

AD is categorized, according to biochemical and clinical changes, into three different stages: pre-clinical i.e., early asymptomatic, mild cognitive impairment (MCI), and eventual dementia [76]. The majority of currently known biomarkers and approaches are focused on the late stages of the illness and may be categorized as follows: (1) neuropsychological tests, (2) neuroimaging techniques, and (3) protein biomarkers in the cerebrospinal fluid (CSF) [25]. Neuropsychological tests include cognitive assessments such as the Mini-Mental State Examination (MMSE) for early diagnosis to track cognitive changes over time and quantify the severity of cognitive impairment; however, this method is limited by factors such as the patient's familiarity with the test and their educational attainment, which limits its sensitivity and specificity [77]. Neuroimaging examinations include fluorodeoxyglucose (FDG)-positron emission tomography (PET) and magnetic resonance imaging (MRI) for monitoring functional abnormalities as well as pathophysiological alterations such as medial temporal lobe atrophy and metabolic problems that can develop without evident cognitive impairment. Though this approach is viable, it has significant time and expense constraints. There are just a few laboratories that provide neuroimaging examinations. As a result, only a limited proportion of patients have access to neuroimaging [78]. Currently, protein biomarkers are the best biomarkers for monitoring AD and clinical research. They include $A\beta1$–40, $A\beta1$–4, phosphorylated tau (ptau), and total tau (t-tau) proteins in the CSF. However, a lumbar puncture is required to get CSF, which is invasive and not well tolerated by patients [78]. The identification of disease-causing genes is also a viable option. Simple, efficient, and inexpensive biomarkers for AD diagnosis are still lacking, especially in the early stages of the illness [25]. Several pieces of literature have found that particular miRNA species found in the biofluid of Alzheimer's patients correlate with clinical alterations [22, 79–81]. Thus, miRNA emerges as a potential biomarker for initial diagnosis of AD as they are present in circulatory fluids which include CSF, seminal fluid, peritoneal fluid, amniotic fluid, pleural fluid, bronchial secretions seminal fluid, serum, plasma, and various other biological fluids [82, 83]. Circulatory miRNAs are a possible diagnostic biomarker for the illness because of their consistency and large quantity. miRNAs are when enwrapped in liposomes or attached to lipoproteins in the CSF, serum, or plasma, they are more stable and may endure harsh environmental conditions [84]. Furthermore, miRNAs may be acquired and measured with ease utilizing real-time PCR, next-generation sequencing (NGS), or microarray. Bio-molecules found in biological fluids such as CSF, tear, urine, and blood are being studied for their possible role in detecting disease progression in Alzheimer's patients. According to previous research, miRNA is a modulator of the pathogenic state exhibited in AD [85]. Several miRNAs like miR-26b [54], miR-34a/c, miR125b, miR-210, and miR-146b are shown to change in blood and brain in Alzheimer's patients, although the direction of changes is not always consistent between both

| Target | miRNA | Function | Bio-fluids | Upregulation (Up) or Downregulation (Down) | References |
|---|---|---|---|---|---|
| APP | miR-106b | Regulate APP expression | Serum | Up | [33, 88, 89] |
|  | miR-101 | Negative regulator of APP expression | Serum | Up | [36, 89, 90] |
|  | miR-16 | Decreased expression of miR-16 lead to accumulation of APP protein in AD | Blood | Up | [37, 91] |
| ADAM10 | miR-23a | Non-amyloidogenic APP processing | Serum | Up | [92, 93] |
|  | miR-107 |  | Plasma | Down | [41, 94] |
|  | miR-451 |  | Plasma-derived extracellular vesicles | Down | [93, 95] |
| BACE1 | miR-9 | TNF-$\alpha$,ephrin-A2 and APP cleavage | CSF exosomes | Up | [96–99] |
|  |  |  | Serum |  |  |
|  | miR-107 |  | Plasma | Down | [41, 94] |
|  | miR-29a |  | Serum | Up | [39, 96, 100] |
|  |  |  | CSF |  |  |
|  | miR-29b |  | Serum | Up | [39, 96, 101] |
|  |  |  | CSF | Down |  |
| BDNF | miR-206 | Growth factor involved in synapse maturation | Serum and plasma | Up | [102–104] |
| CREB1 | miR-134 | Transcription factor involved in synaptic plasticity | Plasma | Up | [105, 106] |
| DLG4 | miR-125a | Scaffold protein (PSD-95) | CSF and Serum | Up | [107, 108] |
| DPYSL2 | miR-181c | Axon guidance (CRMP-2) | Plasma | Up | [86, 98, 109] |
|  |  |  | Serum | Down | [96] |
| EFNA3 | miR-210 | (Ephrin-A3) Axon guidance | Plasma | Up | [86, 110] |

| Target | miRNA | Function | Bio-fluids | Upregulation (Up) or Downregulation (Down) | References |
|---|---|---|---|---|---|
| GRIA1 | miR-137 | Synaptic transmission | Serum | Down | [96, 111] |
| | miR-501 | | Serum | Down | [78, 112] |
| GRIA2 | miR-181a | Neurotransmitter release | Blood | Up | [113, 114] |
| GRIN2A | miR-125b | Synaptic transmission | CSF and Serum | Down | [115–117] |
| GRIN2B | miR-34a | Synaptic transmission | Plasma | Up | [101, 118, 119] |
| | | | CSF | Down | |
| IGF1 | miR-26b | Growth factor involved in synapse maturation | Serum | Up | [116, 120, 121] |
| | | | Blood | | |
| MME (NEP) | miR-26b | Neurite outgrowth | Serum | Up | [116, 121, 122] |
| | | | Blood | | |
| SYN | miR-106b | Inhibit tau phosphorylation | Serum | Up | [88, 89, 123] |
| STIM2 | miR-128 | NMDA-evoked intracellular Ca$^{2+}$ | Plasma | Up | [105, 124, 125] |
| SIRT1 | miR-132 | Acetylation of substrates related to learning and memory | Serum | Dow | [93, 102] |
| SYT1 | miR-146a | Trafficking/neurotransmitter release | Blood | Up | [21, 113, 126] |
| | | | CSF and plasma | Down | [101] |
| TMOD2 | miR-191 | Actin filament organization | Plasma | Down | [127, 128] |
| VAMP2 | miR-34c | Neurotransmitter release Vesicle | Plasma | Up | [129, 130] |

**Table 1.**
*Changes in the level of MiRNAs in the blood, plasma/serum and cerebral-spinal fluid (CSF) of AD patients with their targets and functions.*

miRNA sources [22, 86]. Furthermore, miRNA isolated from Alzheimer's patients' blood plasma and serum including miR-545-3p, miR-107, miR-15b-5p, miR-191-5p has been expected as potential AD biomarkers [22]. MiR-455-3p has emerged as a possible AD biomarker since growing levels in serum are commensurate with levels in AD brains, fibroblasts, lymphocytes, and even AD transgenic models [87]. This emerges the need to further explore the potential of a single miRNA to identify prodromal AD. A panel of miRNAs implicated in pathological processes underlying AD, such as neuroinflammation, has emerged as a diagnostic tool for AD prediction. While much work is being done on miRNA-based biomarkers for AD, few studies in the area have looked at the link between AD biomarkers and synaptic function modulation. **Table 1** summarizes the most important findings in synaptic-related miRNAs obtained from circulating biofluids of AD patients and their potential value as biomarkers. The majority of studies have been done in blood samples, including serum and plasma, indicating a desire to investigate less invasive biomarkers. Certain studies reported earlier demonstrated that reproducibility between studies might be challenging even when miRNAs are obtained from the same sample source. As an example, the drop in miR-132 in serum from mild cognitive impairment (MCI) and AD patients [102, 107], has been replicated in plasma sample [131], although Sheinerman and team found an increase in MCI individuals [105], MiR-132, along with miR-206, which is similarly downregulated in MCI serum, has been proposed as part of a serum-based signature for MCI identification [102]. The adoption of miRNA-based signatures, which take into account the simultaneous modification of many miRNAs, can result in greater accuracy, sensitivity, and specificity values, which could be beneficial for future diagnostic tools. Another signature based on serum-miRNA levels, including synaptic-related miR-23a, miR-29a, and miR-125b has shown promising results in distinguishing Alzheimer's patients from healthy cognitive controls (HCC) [92]. Although results are inconsistent between researches, the diagnostic usefulness of the miR-29a/b family has been examined in serum and CSF [39, 92, 96, 100, 132]. The modification of these miRNAs in biological fluids during AD pathology appears to be obvious. MiR-125b and miR-23a, on the other hand, have continuously increased in serum, demonstrating a strong ability to differentiate between AD and control participants [92, 115]. MiR-125b's potential has also been investigated in CSF, where it has subsequently been offered as a specialized tool [116]. As previously reported, an increase in associated miR-125a levels has been seen in CSF from AD patients, suggesting that it might be used as a biomarker [100, 107]. Limited literature has looked at miRNA levels over time to see whether they might predict the development of MCI into AD. Beneficial diagnostic tool for classify MCI from AD include miR-206 [103], miR-146a, and miR-181a [113], miR-181c [88, 92], miR-181a and miR-181c [105], miR-92a-3p, and miR-210-3p [86], miR-107 [133].

The potential utility and benefits of miRNAs as early biomarkers for AD underscore the urgent need for protocol standardization as a critical tool for accelerating development in generating more accurate findings and bringing breakthroughs to the clinics. Molecular diagnostics companies like DiamiR are already developing and commercializing miRNA-based technologies, demonstrating the progress made in the field and the real possibilities of using miRNAs as biomarkers for AD not only in screening and diagnosis but also as a useful tool for bettering the condition of clinical trial participants.

## 7. Conclusion

MiRNAs play an important role in the progression of AD. Alzheimer's investigation indicates that miRNA may assist to gene regulation, protein-protein expressions, and phenotypic changes in diseases condition and some indication shows that aberrant regulation of miRNA-dependent genes are related to some cellular and molecular events which are liable for Aβ production, neurodegeneration, and NFTs formation. This review highlights the involvement of miRNAs in the regulation of APP expression, BACE1 expression and Aβ clearance. Thus, miRNA is possibly used as a treatment tool for AD. In addition to the therapeutic tool, microRNAs are also emerging as diagnostic tools because of their high sensitivity, efficiency, and specificity. It is found in biological fluids like CSF, extracellular fluid, pleural fluid, seminal fluid, bronchial secretions, breastmilk, serum, blood, plasma, etc. Thus, given the intricacy of AD development, illness history, and diagnosis, future treatment methods such as miRNA and anti-miRNA (antimiR, antagomir) techniques are needed:

i. It will be coupled with improvements in the development of sensitive and precise neuroimaging and biofluid-based diagnostic tools for miRNA and other AD-relevant biomarkers,

ii. It will need to be simultaneous and multimodal, addressing numerous disease pathways, and neurological symptoms to block basic illness progression while minimizing ancillary off-target consequences,

iii. It will be used for screening in conjunction with basic medical care and as a second level diagnostic work-up for expert diagnosis and clinical treatment,

iv. It may entail correct medication therapy and distinct therapeutic development within the neurophysiological perspectives and the systems biology.

## Conflict of interest

The authors declare no conflict of interest.

## Abbreviations

| | |
|---|---|
| 3'UTR | 3'-untranslated region |
| AChE | acetylcholinesterase |
| ACID | APP intracellular domain |
| AD | Alzheimer's disease |
| ADAM10 | a disintegrin and metalloproteinase 10 |
| Ago | argonaute protein |
| AKT | protein kinase B |
| APP | amyloid precursor protein |
| Aβ | amyloid beta |
| BACE1 | β-site amyloid precursor protein cleaving enzyme 1 |
| BDMs | blood-derived monocytes |
| C83 | proteolytic products of APP |
| CCL2/CCR2 | chemokine (c-c motif) ligand 2/chemokine (c-c) receptor type 2 |
| CREB1 | CAMP responsive element binding protein 1 |
| CSF | cerebrospinal fluid |
| DGCR8 | DiGeorge syndrome critical region 8 |
| DLG4 | discs large homolog 4 |
| DPYSL2 | dihydropyrimidinase-related protein 2 |

| | |
|---|---|
| Drosha | ribonuclease III enzyme |
| DUSP6 | dual specificity phosphatase 6 |
| EFNA3 | ephrin A3 |
| Evs | extracellular vesicles |
| FDG | fluorodeoxyglucose |
| FTD | frontotemporal disorder |
| GRIA1 | glutamate receptor 1 |
| GRIN2B | glutamate receptor ionotropic, NMDA 2B |
| GSK-3b | glycogen synthase kinase-3$\beta$ |
| hATTR | hereditary transthyretin-mediated amyloidosis |
| HCC | healthy cognitive controls |
| HEK293 | human embryonic kidney cell-line |
| Ho-1 | heme oxygenase 1 |
| IGF1 | insulin-like growth factor 1 |
| MAPK | mitogen-activated protein kinases |
| MCI | mild cognition impairment |
| MEF2D | myocyte-specific enhancer factor 2D |
| MME (NEP) | membrane metalloendopeptidase (neutral endopeptidase) |
| MMSE | mini-mental state examination |
| MRI | magnetic resonance imaging |
| mTOR | mammalian target of rapamycin |
| N2a | neuro-2-a cell |
| NF-k$\beta$ | nuclear factor kappa beta |
| NFTs | neurofibrillary tangles |
| NGS | next-generation sequencing |
| Nrf2 | nuclear factor erythroid 2-related factor 2 |
| PET | positron emission tomography |
| PPAR | peroxisome proliferator- activated receptor gamma |
| PPP1CA | PP1-alpha catalytic subunit gene |
| pri-miRNAs | primary miRNAs |
| PTEN | phosphatase and tensin homolog |
| RARA | retinoic acid receptor alpha |
| RISC | RNA-induced silencing complex |
| ROCK1 | Rho-associated, coiled-coil-containing protein kinase 1 |
| SAD | sporadic Alzheimer's disease |
| SAMP8 | senescence-accelerated mouse prone |
| sAPP | soluble amyloid precursor protein |
| SH-SY5Y | human derived neuroblastoma cell line |
| siRNA | small interfering RNAs |
| SIRT1 | silent mating type information regulation 2 homolog |
| STIM2 | stromal interaction molecule 2 |
| SYN2 | synapsin II |
| SYT1 | synaptotagmin-1 |
| TMOD2 | tropomodulin 2 |
| TNFAIP1 | TNF alpha induce protein 1 |
| VAMP2 | vesicle-associated membrane protein 2 |

## Author details

Heena Chauhan[1], Pawan Gupta[2] and Bhagawati Saxena[1*]

1 Department of Pharmacology, Institute of Pharmacy, Nirma University, Ahmedabad, India

2 Department of Pharmacology, Shree SK Patel College of Pharmaceutical Education and Research, Ganpat University, Mehsana, India

*Address all correspondence to: bsaxenapharm@gmail.com; bhagawati.saxena@nirmauni.ac.in

IntechOpen

## References

[1] Bekris LM, Yu CE, Bird TD, Tsuang DW. Genetics of Alzheimer disease. Journal of Geriatric Psychiatry and Neurology. 2010;**23**(4):213-227. DOI: 10.1177/0891988710383571

[2] Goedert M, Spillantini MG. Tau mutations in frontotemporal dementia FTDP-17 and their relevance for Alzheimer's disease. Biochimica et Biophysica Acta (BBA)-Molecular Basis of Disease. 2000;**1502**(1):110-121

[3] Dermaut B, Kumar-Singh S, Rademakers R, Theuns J, Cruts M, Van Broeckhoven C. Tau is central in the genetic Alzheimer–frontotemporal dementia spectrum. Trends in Genetics. 2005;**21**(12):664-672

[4] Chavali VD, Agarwal M, Vyas VK, Saxena B. Neuroprotective effects of ethyl Pyruvate against aluminum chloride-induced Alzheimer's disease in rats via inhibiting toll-like receptor 4. Journal of Molecular Neuroscience. 2020;**70**(6):836-850

[5] Tarawneh R, Holtzman DM. The clinical problem of symptomatic Alzheimer disease and mild cognitive impairment. Cold Spring Harbor Perspectives in Medicine. 2012;**2**(5): a006148. DOI: 10.1101/cshperspect. a006148

[6] Sosa-Ortiz AL, Acosta-Castillo I, Prince MJ. Epidemiology of dementias and Alzheimer's disease. Archives of Medical Research. 2012;**43**(8):600-608

[7] Robinson M, Lee BY, Hane FT. Recent progress in Alzheimer's disease research, part 2: Genetics and epidemiology. Journal of Alzheimer's Disease. 2017;**57**(2):317-330. DOI: 10.3233/JAD-161149

[8] Wong W. Economic burden of Alzheimer disease and managed care considerations. The American Journal of Managed Care. 2020;**26**(Suppl. 8): S177-S183

[9] Brookmeyer R, Johnson E, Ziegler-Graham K, Arrighi HM. Forecasting the global burden of Alzheimer's disease. Alzheimer's & Dementia. 2007;**3**(3):186-191

[10] Rajmohan R, Reddy PH. Amyloid-beta and phosphorylated tau accumulations cause abnormalities at synapses of Alzheimer's disease neurons. Journal of Alzheimer's Disease. 2017;**57**(4):975-999. DOI: 10.3233/JAD-160612

[11] Saxena B, Chavali VD. The role of toll like receptor 4 in pathogenesis of Alzheimer's disease induced by aluminum chloride. International Journal of Emerging Technologies and Innovative Research. 2019;**6**(4):96-99

[12] Tiwari S, Atluri V, Kaushik A, Yndart A, Nair M. Alzheimer's disease: Pathogenesis, diagnostics, and therapeutics. International Journal of Nanomedicine. 2019;**14**:5541

[13] Nhan HS, Chiang K, Koo EH. The multifaceted nature of amyloid precursor protein and its proteolytic fragments: Friends and foes. Acta Neuropathologica. 2015;**129**(1):1-19

[14] Coronel R, Palmer C, Bernabeu-Zornoza A, Monteagudo M, Rosca A, Zambrano A, et al. Physiological effects of amyloid precursor protein and its derivatives on neural stem cell biology and signaling pathways involved. Neural Regeneration Research. 2019;**14**(10): 1661

[15] Kim J, Onstead L, Randle S, Price R, Smithson L, Zwizinski C, et al. Aβ40 inhibits amyloid deposition in vivo. Journal of Neuroscience. 2007;**27**(3): 627-633

[16] Sun X, Chen W-D, Wang Y-D. β-Amyloid: The key peptide in the pathogenesis of Alzheimer's disease. Frontiers in Pharmacology. 2015;**6**:221

[17] Zhang C, Khandelwal PJ, Chakraborty R, Cuellar TL, Sarangi S, Patel SA, et al. An AICD-based functional screen to identify APP metabolism regulators. Molecular Neurodegeneration. 2007;**2**(1):1-19

[18] Ballatore C, Lee VM-Y, Trojanowski JQ. Tau-mediated neurodegeneration in Alzheimer's disease and related disorders. Nature Reviews Neuroscience. 2007;**8**(9): 663-672

[19] Lindwall G, Cole RD. Phosphorylation affects the ability of tau protein to promote microtubule assembly. Journal of Biological Chemistry. 1984;**259**(8):5301-5305

[20] Iqbal K, Alonso AC, Chen S, Chohan MO, El-Akkad E, Gong C-X, et al. Tau pathology in Alzheimer disease and other tauopathies. Biochimica et Biophysica Acta (BBA)-Molecular Basis of Disease. 2005; **1739**(2-3):198-210

[21] Angelucci F, Cechova K, Valis M, Kuca K, Zhang B, Hort J. MicroRNAs in Alzheimer's disease: Diagnostic markers or therapeutic agents? Frontiers in Pharmacology. 2019;**10**:665

[22] Swarbrick S, Wragg N, Ghosh S, Stolzing A. Systematic review of miRNA as biomarkers in Alzheimer's disease. Molecular Neurobiology. 2019;**56**(9):6156-6167

[23] O'Brien J, Hayder H, Zayed Y, Peng C. Overview of microRNA biogenesis, mechanisms of actions, and circulation. Frontiers in Endocrinology. 2018;**9**:402

[24] Abe M, Bonini NM. MicroRNAs and neurodegeneration: Role and

impact. Trends in Cell Biology. 2013;**23**(1):30-36

[25] Wei W, Wang Z-Y, Ma L-N, Zhang T-T, Cao Y, Li H. MicroRNAs in Alzheimer's disease: Function and potential applications as diagnostic biomarkers. Frontiers in Molecular Neuroscience. 2020;**13**:160

[26] Long JM, Holtzman DM. Alzheimer disease: An update on pathobiology and treatment strategies. Cell. 2019;**179**(2): 312-339

[27] Yang P, Sun F. Aducanumab: The first targeted Alzheimer's therapy. Drug Discoveries & Therapeutics. 2021;**15**(3):166-168

[28] Ha T-Y. MicroRNAs in human diseases: From cancer to cardiovascular disease. Immune Network. 2011; **11**(3):135-154

[29] Lekka E, Hall J. Noncoding RNAs in disease. FEBS Letters. 2018;**592**(17): 2884-2900

[30] Junn E, Mouradian MM. MicroRNAs in neurodegenerative diseases and their therapeutic potential. Pharmacology & Therapeutics. 2012;**133**(2):142-150

[31] Lau P, De Strooper B. Dysregulated microRNAs in neurodegenerative disorders. Seminars in Cell & Developmental Biology. 2010; **21**(7):768-773

[32] Bazrgar M, Khodabakhsh P, Mohagheghi F, Prudencio M, Ahmadiani A. Brain microRNAs dysregulation: Implication for missplicing and abnormal post-translational modifications of tau protein in Alzheimer's disease and related tauopathies. Pharmacological Research. 2020;**155**:104729

[33] Hébert SS, Horré K, Nicolaï L, Bergmans B, Papadopoulou AS,

Delacourte A, et al. MicroRNA regulation of Alzheimer's amyloid precursor protein expression. Neurobiology of Disease. 2009;**33**(3): 422-428

[34] Kou X, Chen D, Chen N. The regulation of microRNAs in Alzheimer's disease. Frontiers in Neurology. 2020;**11**:288

[35] Thomas L, Florio T, Perez-Castro C. Extracellular vesicles loaded miRNAs as potential modulators shared between glioblastoma, and Parkinson's and Alzheimer's diseases. Frontiers in Cellular Neuroscience. 2020;**14**:360

[36] Vilardo E, Barbato C, Ciotti M, Cogoni C, Ruberti F. MicroRNA-101 regulates amyloid precursor protein expression in hippocampal neurons. Journal of Biological Chemistry. 2010;**285**(24):18344-18351

[37] Liu W, Liu C, Zhu J, Shu P, Yin B, Gong Y, et al. MicroRNA-16 targets amyloid precursor protein to potentially modulate Alzheimer's-associated pathogenesis in SAMP8 mice. Neurobiology of Aging. 2012;**33**(3): 522-534

[38] Long JM, Ray B, Lahiri DK. MicroRNA-153 physiologically inhibits expression of amyloid-β precursor protein in cultured human fetal brain cells and is dysregulated in a subset of Alzheimer disease patients. Journal of Biological Chemistry. 2012;**287**(37): 31298-31310

[39] Hébert SS, Horré K, Nicolaï L, Papadopoulou AS, Mandemakers W, Silahtaroglu AN, et al. Loss of microRNA cluster miR-29a/b-1 in sporadic Alzheimer's disease correlates with increased BACE1/β-secretase expression. Proceedings of the National Academy of Sciences. 2008;**105**(17): 6415-6420

[40] Lei X, Lei L, Zhang Z, Zhang Z, Cheng Y. Downregulated miR-29c correlates with increased BACE1 expression in sporadic Alzheimer's disease. International Journal of Clinical and Experimental Pathology. 2015;**8**(2):1565

[41] Wang W-X, Rajeev BW, Stromberg AJ, Ren N, Tang G, Huang Q, et al. The expression of microRNA miR-107 decreases early in Alzheimer's disease and may accelerate disease progression through regulation of β-site amyloid precursor protein-cleaving enzyme 1. Journal of Neuroscience. 2008;**28**(5):1213-1223

[42] Parsi S, Smith PY, Goupil C, Dorval V, Hébert SS. Preclinical evaluation of miR-15/107 family members as multifactorial drug targets for Alzheimer's disease. Molecular Therapy-Nucleic Acids. 2015;**4**:e256

[43] Shu B, Zhang X, Du G, Fu Q, Huang L. MicroRNA-107 prevents amyloid-β-induced neurotoxicity and memory impairment in mice. International Journal of Molecular Medicine. 2018;**41**(3):1665-1672

[44] Boissonneault V, Plante I, Rivest S, Provost P. MicroRNA-298 and microRNA-328 regulate expression of mouse β-amyloid precursor protein-converting enzyme 1. Journal of Biological Chemistry. 2009;**284**(4): 1971-1981

[45] Liu C-G, Wang J-l, Li L, Xue L-X, Zhang Y-Q, Wang P-C. MicroRNA-135a and-200b, potential biomarkers for Alzheimer's disease, regulate β secretase and amyloid precursor protein. Brain Research. 2014;**1583**: 55-64

[46] Zhang Y, Xing H, Guo S, Zheng Z, Wang H, Xu D. MicroRNA-135b has a neuroprotective role via targeting of β-site APP-cleaving enzyme 1. Experimental and Therapeutic Medicine. 2016;**12**(2):809-814

[47] Kim J, Yoon H, Chung D, Brown JL, Belmonte KC, Kim J. miR-186 is decreased in aged brain and suppresses BACE 1 expression. Journal of Neurochemistry. 2016;**137**(3):436-445

[48] Zhu H-C, Wang L-M, Wang M, Song B, Tan S, Teng J-F, et al. MicroRNA-195 downregulates Alzheimer's disease amyloid-$\beta$ production by targeting BACE1. Brain Research Bulletin. 2012;**88**(6):596-601

[49] Long JM, Ray B, Lahiri DK. MicroRNA-339-5p down-regulates protein expression of $\beta$-site amyloid precursor protein-cleaving enzyme 1 (BACE1) in human primary brain cultures and is reduced in brain tissue specimens of Alzheimer disease subjects. Journal of Biological Chemistry. 2014;**289**(8):5184-5198

[50] Tiribuzi R, Crispoltoni L, Porcellati S, Di Lullo M, Florenzano F, Pirro M, et al. miR128 up-regulation correlates with impaired amyloid $\beta$ (1-42) degradation in monocytes from patients with sporadic Alzheimer's disease. Neurobiology of Aging. 2014;**35**(2):345-356

[51] Zhao Y, Jaber V, Lukiw WJ. Over-expressed pathogenic miRNAs in Alzheimer's disease (AD) and prion disease (PrD) drive deficits in TREM2-mediated A$\beta$42 peptide clearance. Frontiers in Aging Neuroscience. 2016;**8**:140

[52] Guedes JR, Santana I, Cunha C, Duro D, Almeida MR, Cardoso AM, et al. MicroRNA deregulation and chemotaxis and phagocytosis impairment in Alzheimer's disease. Alzheimer's & Dementia: Diagnosis, Assessment & Disease Monitoring. 2016;**3**:7-17

[53] He D, Tan JZ, J. miR-137 attenuates A$\beta$-induced neurotoxicity through inactivation of NF-κB pathway by targeting TNFAIP1 in Neuro2a cells. Biochemical and Biophysical Research Communications. 2017;**490**(3):941-947

[54] Absalon S, Kochanek DM, Raghavan V, Krichevsky AM. MiR-26b, upregulated in Alzheimer's disease, activates cell cycle entry, tau-phosphorylation, and apoptosis in postmitotic neurons. Journal of Neuroscience. 2013;**33**(37):14645-14659

[55] Banzhaf-Strathmann J, Benito E, May S, Arzberger T, Tahirovic S, Kretzschmar H, et al. Micro RNA-125b induces tau hyperphosphorylation and cognitive deficits in Alzheimer's disease. The EMBO Journal. 2014;**33**(15): 1667-1680

[56] Ma X, Liu L, Meng J. MicroRNA-125b promotes neurons cell apoptosis and Tau phosphorylation in Alzheimer's disease. Neuroscience Letters. 2017;**661**:57-62

[57] Wang X, Tan L, Lu Y, Peng J, Zhu Y, Zhang Y, et al. MicroRNA-138 promotes tau phosphorylation by targeting retinoic acid receptor alpha. FEBS Letters. 2015;**589**(6):726-729

[58] Wang G, Huang Y, Wang L-L, Zhang Y-F, Xu J, Zhou Y, et al. MicroRNA-146a suppresses ROCK1 allowing hyperphosphorylation of tau in Alzheimer's disease. Scientific Reports. 2016;**6**(1):1-12

[59] Wang Y, Veremeyko T, Wong AH-K, El Fatimy R, Wei Z, Cai W, et al. Downregulation of miR-132/212 impairs S-nitrosylation balance and induces tau phosphorylation in Alzheimer's disease. Neurobiology of Aging. 2017;**51**:156-166

[60] Luigetti M, Romano A, Di Paolantonio A, Bisogni G, Sabatelli M. Diagnosis and treatment of hereditary transthyretin amyloidosis (hATTR) polyneuropathy: Current perspectives on improving patient care. Therapeutics and Clinical Risk Management. 2020;**16**:109

[61] Laina A, Gatsiou A, Georgiopoulos G, Stamatelopoulos K, Stellos K. RNA therapeutics in cardiovascular precision medicine. Frontiers in Physiology. 2018;**9**:953

[62] Li Z, Rana TM. Therapeutic targeting of microRNAs: Current status and future challenges. Nature Reviews Drug Discovery. 2014;**13**(8):622-638

[63] Fu J, Peng L, Tac T, Chen Y, Li Z, Li J. Regulatory roles of the miR-200 family in neurodegenerative diseases. Biomedicine & Pharmacotherapy. 2019;**119**:109409

[64] Higaki S, Muramatsu M, Matsuda A, Matsumoto K, Satoh J-i, Michikawa M, et al. Defensive effect of microRNA-200b/c against amyloid-beta peptide-induced toxicity in Alzheimer's disease models. PLoS One. 2018;**13**(5):e0196929

[65] Tramutola A, Triplett JC, Di Domenico F, Niedowicz DM, Murphy MP, Coccia R, et al. Alteration of mTOR signaling occurs early in the progression of Alzheimer disease (AD): Analysis of brain from subjects with pre-clinical AD, amnestic mild cognitive impairment and late-stage AD. Journal of Neurochemistry. 2015;**133**(5):739-749

[66] Zhou Y, Wang ZF, Li W, Hong H, Chen J, Tian Y, et al. Protective effects of microRNA-330 on amyloid β-protein production, oxidative stress, and mitochondrial dysfunction in Alzheimer's disease by targeting VAV1 via the MAPK signaling pathway. Journal of Cellular Biochemistry. 2018;**119**(7):5437-5448

[67] Li J, Wang H. miR-15b reduces amyloid-β accumulation in SH-SY5Y cell line through targetting NF-κB signaling and BACE1. Bioscience Reports. 2018;**38**(6):BSR20180051

[68] Fang M, Wang J, Zhang X, Geng Y, Hu Z, Rudd JA, et al. The miR-124 regulates the expression of BACE1/β-secretase correlated with cell death in Alzheimer's disease. Toxicology Letters. 2012;**209**(1):94-105

[69] An F, Gong G, Wang Y, Bian M, Yu L, Wei C. MiR-124 acts as a target for Alzheimer's disease by regulating BACE1. Oncotarget. 2017;**8**(69):114065

[70] Santa-Maria I, Alaniz ME, Renwick N, Cela C, Fulga TA, Van Vactor D, et al. Dysregulation of microRNA-219 promotes neurodegeneration through post-transcriptional regulation of tau. The Journal of Clinical Investigation. 2015;**125**(2):681-686

[71] Zhang Y, Li Q, Liu C, Gao S, Ping H, Wang J, et al. MiR-214-3p attenuates cognition defects via the inhibition of autophagy in SAMP8 mouse model of sporadic Alzheimer's disease. Neurotoxicology. 2016;**56**:139-149

[72] Han L, Zhou Y, Zhang R, Wu K, Lu Y, Li Y, et al. MicroRNA let-7f-5p promotes bone marrow mesenchymal stem cells survival by targeting caspase-3 in Alzheimer disease model. Frontiers in Neuroscience. 2018;**12**:333

[73] Geng L, Zhang T, Liu W, Chen Y. Inhibition of miR-128 abates Aβ-mediated cytotoxicity by targeting PPAR-γ via NF-κB inactivation in primary mouse cortical neurons and Neuro2a cells. Yonsei Medical Journal. 2018;**59**(9):1096-1106

[74] Kou X, Chen N. Resveratrol as a natural autophagy regulator for prevention and treatment of Alzheimer's disease. Nutrients. 2017;**9**(9):927

[75] Song Y, Wang X, Wang X, Wang J, Hao Q, Hao J, et al. Osthole-loaded nanoemulsion enhances brain target in the treatment of Alzheimer's disease via intranasal administration. Oxidative

Medicine and Cellular Longevity. 2021;**2021**:8844455

[76] Croisile B, Auriacombe S, Etcharry-Bouyx F, Vercelletto M. Les nouvelles recommandations 2011 du National Institute on Aging et de l'Alzheimer's Association sur le diagnostic de la maladie d'Alzheimer : Stades précliniques, mild cognitive impairment et démence. Revue Neurologique. 2012;**168**(6):471-482

[77] Norris DR, Clark MS, Shipley S. The mental status examination. American Family Physician. 2016;**94**(8):635-641

[78] Hara N, Kikuchi M, Miyashita A, Hatsuta H, Saito Y, Kasuga K, et al. Serum microRNA miR-501-3p as a potential biomarker related to the progression of Alzheimer's disease. Acta Neuropathologica Communications. 2017;**5**(1):1-9

[79] Keller A, Backes C, Haas J, Leidinger P, Maetzler W, Deuschle C, et al. Validating Alzheimer's disease micro RNAs using next-generation sequencing. Alzheimer's & Dementia. 2016;**12**(5):565-576

[80] Takousis P, Sadlon A, Schulz J, Wohlers I, Dobricic V, Middleton L, et al. Differential expression of microRNAs in Alzheimer's disease brain, blood, and cerebrospinal fluid. Alzheimer's & Dementia. 2019;**15**(11): 1468-1477

[81] Wiedrick JT, Phillips JI, Lusardi TA, McFarland TJ, Lind B, Sandau US, et al. Validation of MicroRNA biomarkers for Alzheimer's disease in human cerebrospinal fluid. Journal of Alzheimer's Disease. 2019;**67**(3):875-891

[82] Kumar S, Reddy PH. Are circulating microRNAs peripheral biomarkers for Alzheimer's disease? Biochimica et Biophysica Acta (BBA)-Molecular Basis of Disease. 2016;**1862**(9):1617-1627

[83] Weber JA, Baxter DH, Zhang S, Huang DY, Huang KH, Lee MJ, et al. The microRNA spectrum in 12 body fluids. Clinical Chemistry. 2010;**56**(11): 1733-1741

[84] Van den Berg M, Krauskopf J, Ramaekers J, Kleinjans J, Prickaerts J, Briedé J. Circulating microRNAs as potential biomarkers for psychiatric and neurodegenerative disorders. Progress in Neurobiology. 2020;**185**:101732

[85] Ludwig N, Leidinger P, Becker K, Backes C, Fehlmann T, Pallasch C, et al. Distribution of miRNA expression across human tissues. Nucleic Acids Research. 2016;**44**(8):3865-3877

[86] Siedlecki-Wullich D, Català-Solsona J, Fábregas C, Hernández I, Clarimon J, Lleó A, et al. Altered microRNAs related to synaptic function as potential plasma biomarkers for Alzheimer's disease. Alzheimer's Research & Therapy. 2019;**11**(1):1-11

[87] Kumar S, Reddy AP, Yin X, Reddy PH. Novel MicroRNA-455-3p and its protective effects against abnormal APP processing and amyloid beta toxicity in Alzheimer's disease. Biochimica et Biophysica Acta (BBA)-Molecular Basis of Disease. 2019;**1865**(9):2428-2440

[88] Guo R, Fan G, Zhang J, Wu C, Du Y, Ye H, et al. A 9-microRNA signature in serum serves as a noninvasive biomarker in early diagnosis of Alzheimer's disease. Journal of Alzheimer's Disease. 2017;**60**(4):1365-1377. DOI: 10.3233/JAD-170343

[89] Cheng A, Doecke JD, Sharples R, Villemagne VL, Fowler CJ, Rembach A, et al. Prognostic serum miRNA biomarkers associated with Alzheimer's disease shows concordance with neuropsychological and neuroimaging assessment. Molecular Psychiatry. 2015;**20**(10):1188-1196

[90] Long JML, DK. MicroRNA-101 downregulates Alzheimer's amyloid-β precursor protein levels in human cell cultures and is differentially expressed. Biochemical and Biophysical Research Communications. 2011;**404**(4):889-895

[91] Wu HZY, Thalamuthu A, Cheng L, Fowler C, Masters CL, Sachdev P, et al. Differential blood miRNA expression in brain amyloid imaging-defined Alzheimer's disease and controls. Alzheimer's Research & Therapy. 2020;**12**(59):1-11

[92] Barbagallo C, Mostile G, Baglieri G, Giunta F, Luca A, Raciti L, et al. Specific signatures of serum miRNAs as potential biomarkers to discriminate clinically similar neurodegenerative and vascular-related diseases. Cellular and Molecular Neurobiology. 2020;**40**(4):531-546

[93] Siedlecki-Wullich D, Miñano-Molina AJ, Rodríguez-Álvarez J. microRNAs as early biomarkers of Alzheimer's disease: A synaptic perspective. Cells. 2021;**10**(1):113

[94] Wang J, Chen C, Zhang Y. An investigation of microRNA-103 and microRNA-107 as potential blood-based biomarkers for disease risk and progression of Alzheimer's disease. Journal of Clinical Laboratory Analysis. 2020;**34**(1):e23006

[95] Gámez-Valero A, Campdelacreu J, Vilas D, Ispierto L, Reñé R, Álvarez R, et al. Exploratory study on microRNA profiles from plasma-derived extracellular vesicles in Alzheimer's disease and dementia with Lewy bodies. Translational Neurodegeneration. 2019;**8**(1):1-17

[96] Geekiyanage H, Jicha GA, Nelson PT, Chan C. Blood serum miRNA: Non-invasive biomarkers for Alzheimer's disease. Experimental Neurology. 2012;**235**(2):491-496

[97] Riancho J, Vázquez-Higuera JL, Pozueta A, Lage C, Kazimierczak M, Bravo M, et al. MicroRNA profile in patients with Alzheimer's disease: Analysis of miR-9-5p and miR-598 in raw and exosome enriched cerebrospinal fluid samples. Journal of Alzheimer's Disease. 2017;**57**(2):483-491

[98] Schonrock N, Humphreys DT, Preiss T, Götz J. Target gene repression mediated by miRNAs miR-181c and miR-9 both of which are down-regulated by amyloid-β. Journal of Molecular Neuroscience. 2012; **46**(2):324-335

[99] Schonrock N, Ke YD, Humphreys D, Staufenbiel M, Ittner LM, Preiss T, et al. Neuronal microRNA deregulation in response to Alzheimer's disease amyloid-β. PloS One. 2010;**5**(6):e11070

[100] Müller M, Jäkel L, Bruinsma IB, Claassen JA, Kuiperij HB, Verbeek MM. MicroRNA-29a is a candidate biomarker for Alzheimer's disease in cell-free cerebrospinal fluid. Molecular Neurobiology. 2016;**53**(5):2894-2899

[101] Kiko T, Nakagawa K, Tsuduki T, Furukawa K, Arai H, Miyazawa T. MicroRNAs in plasma and cerebrospinal fluid as potential markers for Alzheimer's disease. Journal of Alzheimer's Disease. 2014;**39**(2): 253-259

[102] Xie B, Zhou H, Zhang R, Song M, Yu L, Wang L, et al. Serum miR-206 and miR-132 as potential circulating biomarkers for mild cognitive impairment. Journal of Alzheimer's Disease. 2015;**45**(3):721-731

[103] Kenny A, McArdle H, Calero M, Rabano A, Madden SF, Adamson K, et al. Elevated plasma microRNA-206 levels predict cognitive decline and progression to dementia from mild cognitive impairment. Biomolecules. 2019;**9**(11):734

[104] Lee ST, Chu K, Jung KH, Kim JH, Huh JY, Yoon H, et al. miR-206 regulates brain-derived neurotrophic factor in Alzheimer disease model. Annals of Neurology. 2012;**72**(2):269-277

[105] Sheinerman KS, Tsivinsky VG, Abdullah L, Crawford F, Umansky SR. Plasma microRNA biomarkers for detection of mild cognitive impairment: Biomarker validation study. Aging (Albany NY). 2013;**5**(12):925

[106] Bicker S, Lackinger M, Weiß K, Schratt G. MicroRNA-132,-134, and-138: A microRNA troika rules in neuronal dendrites. Cellular and Molecular Life Sciences. 2014;**71**(20):3987-4005

[107] Denk J, Oberhauser F, Kornhuber J, Wiltfang J, Fassbender K, Schroeter ML, et al. Specific serum and CSF microRNA profiles distinguish sporadic behavioural variant of frontotemporal dementia compared with Alzheimer patients and cognitively healthy controls. PloS One. 2018;**13**(5):e0197329

[108] Muddashetty RS, Nalavadi VC, Gross C, Yao X, Xing L, Laur O, et al. Reversible inhibition of PSD-95 mRNA translation by miR-125a, FMRP phosphorylation, and mGluR signaling. Molecular Cell. 2011;**42**(5):673-688

[109] Zhou H, Zhang R, Lu K, Yu W, Xie B, Cui D, et al. Deregulation of miRNA-181c potentially contributes to the pathogenesis of AD by targeting collapsin response mediator protein 2 in mice. Journal of the Neurological Sciences. 2016;**367**:3-10

[110] Pulkkinen K, Malm T, Turunen M, Koistinaho J, Ylä-Herttuala S. Hypoxia induces microRNA miR-210 in vitro and in vivo: Ephrin-A3 and neuronal pentraxin 1 are potentially regulated by miR-210. FEBS Letters. 2008;**582**(16): 2397-2401

[111] Loohuis NFO, Ba W, Stoerchel PH, Kos A, Jager A, Schratt G, et al. MicroRNA-137 controls AMPA-receptor-mediated transmission and mGluR-dependent LTD. Cell Reports. 2015;**11**(12):1876-1884

[112] Hu Z, Zhao J, Hu T, Luo Y, Zhu JL, Z. miR-501-3p mediates the activity-dependent regulation of the expression of AMPA receptor subunit GluA1. Journal of Cell Biology. 2015;**208**(7): 949-959

[113] Ansari A, Maffioletti E, Milanesi E, Marizzoni M, Frisoni GB, Blin O, et al. miR-146a and miR-181a are involved in the progression of mild cognitive impairment to Alzheimer's disease. Neurobiology of Aging. 2019;**82**:102-109

[114] Rodriguez-Ortiz CJ, Prieto GA, Martini AC, Forner S, Trujillo-Estrada L, LaFerla FM, et al. miR-181a negatively modulates synaptic plasticity in hippocampal cultures and its inhibition rescues memory deficits in a mouse model of Alzheimer's disease. Aging Cell. 2020;**19**(3):e13118

[115] Tan L, Yu J-T, Liu Q-Y, Tan M-S, Zhang W, Hu N, et al. Circulating miR-125b as a biomarker of Alzheimer's disease. Journal of the Neurological Sciences. 2014;**336**(1-2):52-56

[116] Galimberti D, Villa C, Fenoglio C, Serpente M, Ghezzi L, Cioffi SM, et al. Circulating miRNAs as potential biomarkers in Alzheimer's disease. Journal of Alzheimer's Disease. 2014;**42**(4):1261-1267

[117] Edbauer D, Neilson JR, Foster KA, Wang C-F, Seeburg DP, Batterton MN, et al. Regulation of synaptic structure and function by FMRP-associated MicroRNAs miR-125b and miR-132. Neuron. 2010;**65**(3):373-384

[118] Sarkar S, Engler-Chiurazzi E, Cavendish J, Povroznik J, Russell A,

Quintana D, et al. Over-expression of miR-34a induces rapid cognitive impairment and Alzheimer's disease-like pathology. Brain Research. 2019;**1721**:146327

[119] Xu Y, Chen P, Wang X, Yao J, Zhuang S. miR-34a deficiency in APP/PS1 mice promotes cognitive function by increasing synaptic plasticity via AMPA and NMDA receptors. Neuroscience Letters. 2018;**670**:94-104

[120] Liu H, Chu W, Gong L, Gao X, Wang W. MicroRNA-26b is upregulated in a double transgenic mouse model of Alzheimer's disease and promotes the expression of amyloid-β by targeting insulin-like growth factor 1. Molecular Medicine Reports. 2016;**13**(3):2809-2814

[121] Satoh J-i, Kino Y, Niida S. MicroRNA-Seq data analysis pipeline to identify blood biomarkers for Alzheimer's disease from public data. Biomarker Insights. 2015;**10**:21-31

[122] Chu T, Shu Y, Qu Y, Gao S, Zhang L. miR-26b inhibits total neurite outgrowth, promotes cells apoptosis and downregulates neprilysin in Alzheimer's disease. International Journal of Clinical and Experimental Pathology. 2018;**11**(7):3383-3389

[123] Liu W, Zhao J, Lu G. miR-106b inhibits tau phosphorylation at Tyr18 by targeting Fyn in a model of Alzheimer's disease. Biochemical and Biophysical Research Communications. 2016;**478**(2):852-857

[124] Deng M, Zhang Q, Wu Z, Ma T, He A, Zhang T, et al. Mossy cell synaptic dysfunction causes memory imprecision via miR-128 inhibition of STIM2 in Alzheimer's disease mouse model. Aging Cell. 2020;**19**(5):e13144

[125] Sheinerman KS, Tsivinsky VG, Crawford F, Mullan MJ, Abdullah L, Umansky SR. Plasma microRNA biomarkers for detection of mild cognitive impairment. Aging (Albany NY). 2012;**4**(9):590

[126] Prada I, Gabrielli M, Turola E, Iorio A, D'Arrigo G, Parolisi R, et al. Glia-to-neuron transfer of miRNAs via extracellular vesicles: A new mechanism underlying inflammation-induced synaptic alterations. Acta neuropathologica. 2018;**135**(4): 529-550

[127] Hu Z, Yu D, Gu Q-h, Yang Y, Tu K, Zhu J, et al. miR-191 and miR-135 are required for long-lasting spine remodelling associated with synaptic long-term depression. Nature Communications. 2014;**5**(1):1-17

[128] Kumar P, Dezso Z, MacKenzie C, Oestreicher J, Agoulnik S, Byrne M, et al. Circulating miRNA biomarkers for Alzheimer's disease. PloS One. 2013;**8**(7):e69807

[129] Bhatnagar S, Chertkow H, Schipper HM, Shetty V, Yuan Z, Jones T, et al. Increased microRNA-34c abundance in Alzheimer's disease circulating blood plasma. Frontiers in Molecular Neuroscience. 2014;**7**:2

[130] Hu S, Wang H, Chen K, Cheng P, Gao S, Liu J, et al. MicroRNA-34c downregulation ameliorates amyloid-β-induced synaptic failure and memory deficits by targeting VAMP2. Journal of Alzheimer's Disease. 2015;**48**(3):673-686. DOI: 10.3233/JAD-150432

[131] Cha DJ, Mengel D, Mustapic M, Liu W, Selkoe DJ, Kapogiannis D, et al. miR-212 and miR-132 are downregulated in neurally derived plasma exosomes of Alzheimer's patients. Frontiers in Neuroscience. 2019;**13**:1208

[132] Villa C, Ridolfi E, Fenoglio C, Ghezzi L, Vimercati R, Clerici F, et al.

Expression of the transcription factor Sp1 and its regulatory hsa-miR-29b in peripheral blood mononuclear cells from patients with Alzheimer's disease. Journal of Alzheimer's Disease. 2013;**35**(3):487-494

[133] Beccia M, Ceschin V, Bozzao A, Romano A, Biraschi F, Fantozzi L, et al. Headache and visual symptoms in two patients with MRI alterations in posterior cerebral artery territory. Clinical Therapeutics. 2009;**160**(2):125-127

# Perspective Chapter: Exercise-Eating Pattern and Social Inclusion (EES) is an Effective Modulator of Pathophysiological Hallmarks of Alzheimer's Disease

*Afroza Sultana and Md Alauddin*

## Abstract

Alzheimer's Disease (AD), a common type of dementia, characterized by the presence of aggregated extracellular amyloid-beta (Aβ), intracellular hyper phosphorylation of tau protein and neurodegenerative with cognitive decline. It is projected that 141 million people will be suffering with AD by 2050 but no effective drug treatment is discovered without side effects. There is an urgent need for the application of alternative and non-pharmacological interventions for AD. Sporadically found that exercise or diet therapy or social activity may positively influence the AD. In this review we discussed the process of how Exercise-Eating pattern and Social inclusion (EES) has been shown to have fewer side effects and better adherence with AD. In this mechanism the EES can modulate the brain metabolic factors, brain-derived neurotrophic, ketone bodies, lactate, cathepsin-B, irisin, hormonal balance in AD. This review also described the potential biological mechanisms underlying exercise (modulation of biomolecule turnover, antioxidant and anti inflammation), eating pattern (bioactive compounds) and social inclusion that is very important to ameliorate the pathophysiological hallmarks of Alzheimer's disease. Thus, this EES can be an effective approach to manage the neurodegenerative disorder as well as Alzheimer's disease.

**Keywords:** Exercise-eating pattern and social inclusion (EES), neuromodulators, metabolic factors, pathophysiological-hallmarks, new approach to AD

## 1. Introduction

Alzheimer's disease (AD) is a form of dementia, currently affecting over 55 million people worldwide. This alarming situation is projected to the elevation of 88 million people by 2050 [1, 2]. It is a complex mechanism of neurodegenerative disorder clinically categorized by advanced and continuing deterioration in intellectual capability of the brain and biochemical change due to the presence of neurotic threads, specific areas of the brain function damage subsequently synaptic signal loss. This consequence occurs due to the accumulation of specific protein amyloid-β to the external neurons and modification of the specific tau protein by hyper phosphorylation and ultimately neurofibrillary twists (NFTs) are formed in the neuron cell of the brain. This mechanism is responsible to intellectual deficit, remembrance loss, and then neuron expiry [3, 4]. AD is one of the pathetic disease eases due to the presence of disability in the oldest people and it was found that the prevalence of AD is less than 1% in the people who are underneath 60 years of age, but this prevalence is increasing to 40% among people who are older than 85 [5]. The most important thing is that, there is no specific drug for the treatment of AD to date [4]. The alarming disease burden is concerned in the world, because the projected global population of older adults (defined as those aged >60 year) in the year of 2050 will be 2 billion (approximately 21% of the world's population) out of them 392 million will be over 80 years of old [6]. Presently preventive measures are getting more attention than pharmacological interventions after unsuccessful clinical trials of some promising drugs designed for targeting Aβ and tau proteins. Though, there is no specific treatment of the AD but world scientists are trying to control the gradual growth of AD by multidomain non pharmaceutical intervention such as exercise or diet, and intellectual or physical activity that can prevent cognitive decline at-risk of the oldest population [7]. There is no available information about together-intervention of exercise with diet pattern and social inclusion to ameliorate the prevalence of AD. This is a very important and socially demanding strategy of mass elder people rather than pharmacological intervention.

## 2. Pathological hallmarks of AD

Two most important determinants in or out of the neuron cells in the brain that are involved in the mechanism of dementia progression, i.e., the β-amyloid peptide and tau proteins. The pathophysiological change of AD is normally carried out by measuring the deposition of β-amyloid peptide, a 39–43 amino acid chain that is produced in the brain and organized a flame-shaped neurofibrillary tangles of tau protein in the affected region of the brain [3]. In patient of AD, one of the determinant (β-amyloid peptide) in the brain is found abnormal due to the genetic mutations in the gene of precursor protein of β-amyloid peptide and Presenilins (PS1 and PS2) which lead to anomalous Aβ accumulation outside the neuron in the brain [4]. Another important determinant tau protein treats the microtubule gathering and maintenance due to the hyperphosphorylation of tau protein and is the cause of AD pathology, The actually mechanism of abnormal microtubule gathering is hyper phosphorylation of tau protein because the modified tau protein can accelerate the formation of neurofibrillary tangles (NFTs), that is associated with loss of remembrance and wisdom hearts [8]. The microtubule disassembly (neurofibrillary tangles; NFTs) may likewise found in other distinctive neurodegenerative diseases, have some distinguishing morphological change rather than AD and this is due to a distinctive conformation of tau isoforms that could easily differentiate from AD [9]. On the other hand, the degree of dementia was observed to be weakly correlated with the amounts and distribution of Aβ deposition within the brain [10]. In particular, the increased deposition of Aβ peptide outside the neuron cell can cause abnormal synaptic signal transduction, intellectual linkage, mitochondrial energy transduction, apoptosis of neuronal cell and, ultimately remembrance forfeiture, the hallmark of AD [11, 12]. Even though some neurotoxicity occurs in the neuronal cell, the mechanism of neurotoxicity caused by Aβ is not fully discovered. Although some studies showed that the abnormal accumulation of Aβ peptide in the brain causes induction of oxidative stress and neuroinflammation, the most important cause of neurotoxicity [13]. Early detection of the determinants is one the most important parameters for the management of AD. But the aforementioned two determinants are very difficult to early determination. Thus defective metabolism of glucose in the brain may be

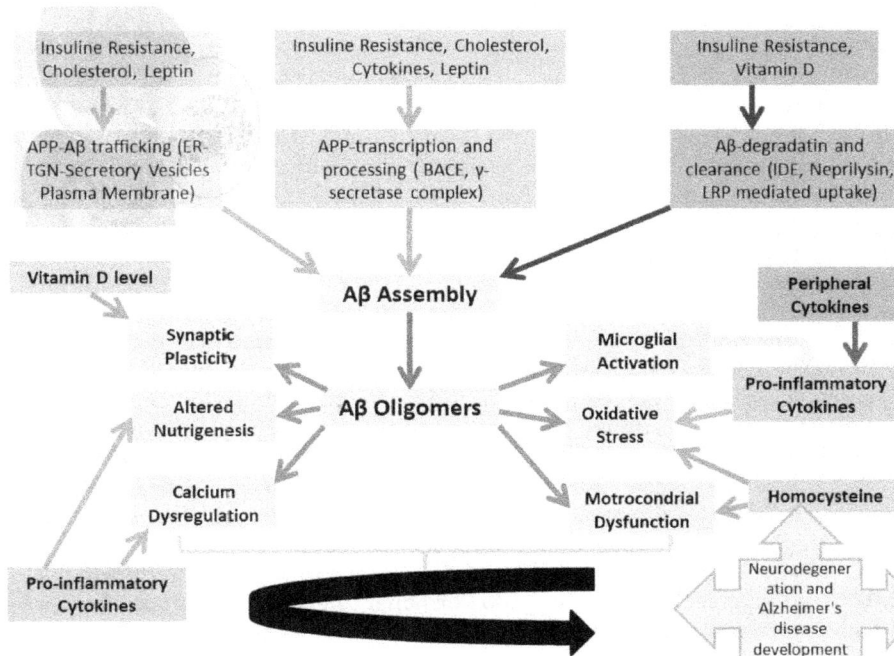

**Figure 1.**
*Various modifiable risk determinants in AD pathology [4].*

one of the earliest hallmarks of AD. The detection of brain glucose hypometabolism is measured by the determination of fluoro-2-deoxy-D-glucose positron emission tomography imaging system. This technique has been suggested as an effective early diagnostic tool for AD. Several studies showed the sensitivity and effectiveness of the brain glucose hypometabolism technique (about 90%) for the early diagnosis of AD [14]. Moreover, amino acids may be another hallmark of AD. For instance, abnormal elevation of homocysteine (Hcy) in the AD population. Studies showed that hyper-homocysteinemia is accompanied with amplified intellectual deterioration in healthy older adults with a higher risk of perceptive deficiency [15]. Another study found that abnormal plasma homocysteine and distressed homocysteine amino acid metabolism are risk factors for intellectual concept [5]. Several potential mechanisms have been studied on the harmful effects of homocysteine amino acid in the brain including oxidative deterioration [16], cerebrovascular impairment [17], DNA destruction [18], and activation of N-methyl-D-aspartate receptors [19]. In the **Figure 1**, we summarized the various modifiable risk determinants that are responsible for AD pathology.

## 3. Mechanisms involved for the development of AD

The Aβ peptide (approximate size ~4 kDa) is resulting by cleavage of the larger β-amyloid precursor protein (AβPP). β- and γ-secretase are the two membrane-bound endoprotease activities sequentially cleaved the AβPP to produce (**Figure 2**) the most abundant fragment Aβ40 (~80 to 90%) and Aβ42 (~5 to 10%). The somewhat extensive forms of Aβ, predominantly Aβ42, is the principal culprit for the deposition in the brain [20]. The enzyme, β-Secretase is a protease which have two major homologous (>65%) forms, one is β-site Amyloid Precursor Protein Cleaving Enzyme (BACE1) and the other is BACE2. The most important Enzyme BACE1 is mainly accountable for β-amyloid peptide production higher in the brain than BACE2 which is mostly present in the peripheral tissues. Animal studies stated that the protease BACE1 is the foremost β-secretase action in the brain, however, some residual motion might be attributable by the BACE2. Besides the brain, The BACE1 are also found in another cell type such as pancreatic β-cells where they are highly expressed in mRNA levels, however, this pancreatic isoform of BACE1 is distinctive from the brain and may not cleave AβPP. It was found that BACE1 action upsurges with oldness and is highly found (two to five-fold) in irregular AD [21, 22]. It is important that the lack of protease activity of BACE1 is related to prevent β-amyloid peptide synthesis [23]. Recent studies also observed that in a suitable situation cathepsin B or cathepsin D may help to serve such kind of enzyme like β-secretase enzymes. The two enzymes, β- and γ-secretase were considered to be the leading goals for the advance of anti-AD medications [24]. For example, alterations in γ-secretase activity by the change of allosteric γ-secretase controlling representatives may prevent the production of β-amyloid peptide [25]. Study showed a reduction in BACE1 expression that is related to glucose metabolism via regulation of insulin mRNA expression. In vivo experiments stated that reduction of BACE1 expression may lower plasma insulin concentrations and body weight through the controlling of regular glucose acceptance and insulin sensitivity [26].

Another relationship of AD has also been exposed to be concomitant with inflammation, glucose metabolism and hormonal balance. For instance, the inflammatory markers have been isolated in the cerebrospinal fluid (CSF) and abnormal amyloid formation found in the brain of AD that is much related to high expression of inflammatory molecules interleukin-6 (IL-6). This relationship is not only found in the brain but also in the other fluid such as the lumbar and ventricular region in patients with AD. Another relationship was found that circulating IL-6 is highly expressed before symptomatic sign of dementia and this increased IL-6 is related with low male hormone like testosterone in older men with type-II diabetes Mellitus (T2DM) and AD [27–29]. It was found that male hormone secretion is hampered by inflammatory molecules IL-6 and this is much

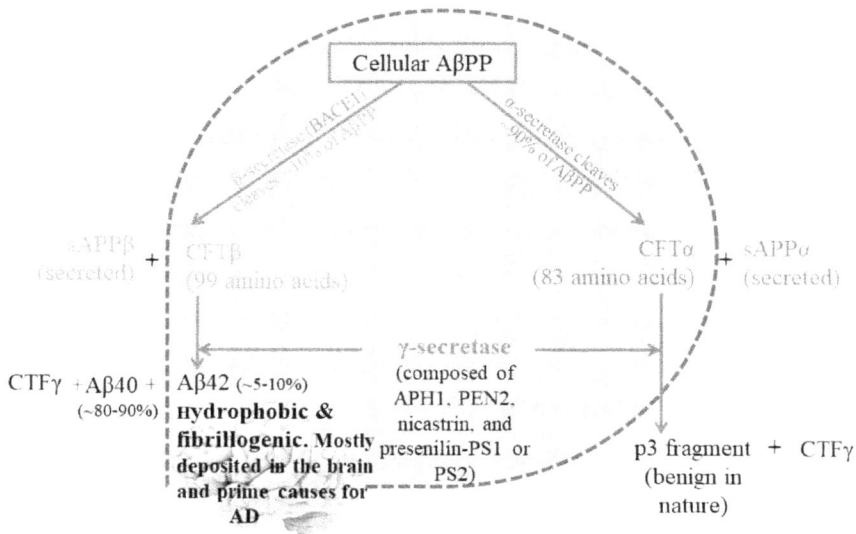

**Figure 2.**
*Amyloidogenic pathway involved for development of AD [32–35].*

related to inflammation and oxidative stress, hormonal imbalance and T2DM with AD pathology [30–31]. **Figure 2** summarized the amyloidogenic pathway involved for development of AD [32–35].

## 4. Mechanisms involved for the prevention of AD

The prevention of AD means the degradation of β-amyloid peptides by enzymes such as Aβ degrading enzyme Neprilysin (NEP) and insulin degrading enzyme (IDE). There are many enzymes, the aforementioned two important enzymes are metalloprotease which are responsible for most of the Aβ degradation [36, 37]. The membrane bound Neprilysin is actually type II metalloprotease which degrades the extracellular variety of peptides but the IDE enzyme can degrade both intra- and extracellular [38]. Though the affinity of IDE enzyme to the insulin is (twenty times higher) higher than Aβ but it hydrolyzes slowly. It is important that the insulin may be responsible for cleavage of β-amyloid peptides, this is the basic mechanism among type II diabetes, hyperinsulinemia, and AD [39, 40]. Most of the Aβ degradation occurs by the influence of NEP, like lysosomal degradation of cathepsin B [41]. Another study stated that other enzymes such as Endothelin Converting Enzyme (ECE), Angiotensin-Converting Enzyme (ACE), and Matrix Metalloproteinase-9 (MMP-9) may also have Aβ degrading properties [42]. Though the substantial degradation of β-amyloid peptides occurs in the brain, their undegraded portion is transported through the blood brain barrier (BBB) into the circulation by specific mechanisms. The soluble part of β-amyloid peptide is switched through the BBB into the abluminal site of the brain by the low-density lipoprotein receptor-related protein (LRP) and into the luminal side of the blood by the receptor for advanced glycation end products (RAGE) [43, 44]. Disturbing this mechanism may cause an increase of Aβ level which may be attached with other widespread co-morbid vascular irregularities in the brain function of AD. This change may exaggerate the development of amyloid pathology [45]. **Figure 3** summarized the detailed preventive mechanism of AD by Aβ degradation pathway. The frequency of AD is found meaningfully higher in women than to men (almost two-thirds) indicating a strong association of sex hormones with the AD [46]. Study observed that testosterone levels are inversely associated with the plasma levels of β-amyloid peptides in elderly men population [47]. Testosterone may provide different neuroprotective effects including enlightening intellectual presentation and synaptic signal transduction by increasing relaxation, modulation synapse density level on the brain hippocampal dendritic spines [48, 49]. This hormone is also important for maintaining hippocampal function in elderly population [50], increasing blood supply to the cerebral and increasing glucose metabolism in the responsive brain regions as well as reduced the aggregation of β-amyloid peptides and neurotoxicity. Testosterone may reducing the tau protein hyperphosphorylation and in vivo experiment showed that the reduction of testosterone is directly associated with reduce intellectual performance, and it could be revised by testosterone supplementation [51, 52]. Women are more prone to AD than men because testosterone is basically a male hormone and most abundant testosterone is converted into estrogen and other adrenal hormones in women. The study showed that women are more prone to AD symptoms due to lack of testosterone [53]. Previous animal study indicated that testosterone (in male) and estrogen (in female) could modulate the invention of β-amyloid peptides by the disturbing of BACE1 action [54, 55]. The hormone like testosterone is an effective modulator of endogenous β-amyloid peptides degrading enzymes such as NEP. Animal study observed that neuronal expression of NEP is enhanced by the action of testosterone which in turn reduces the β-amyloid peptide level and ultimately reduces the symptoms of AD [56]. The increase of β-amyloid peptides degrading enzymes positively

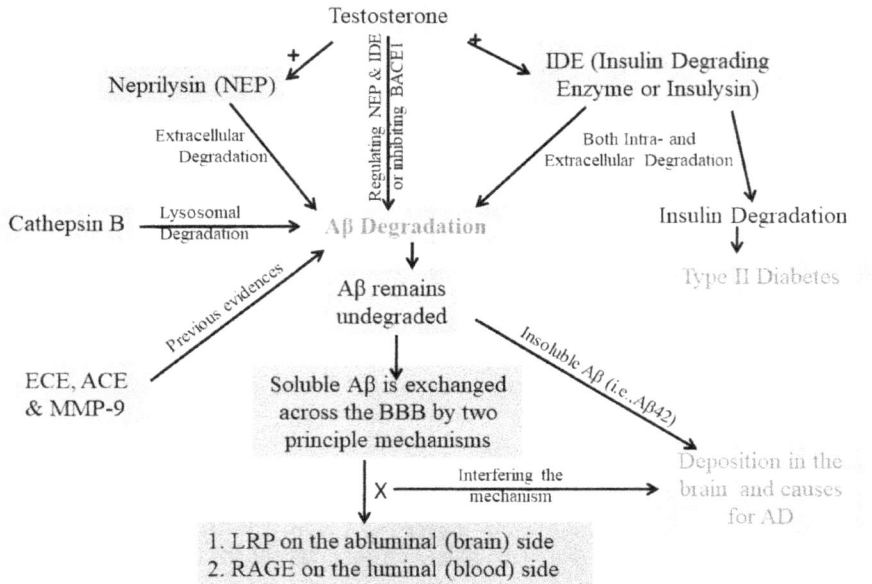

**Figure 3.**
*Preventive mechanism of AD by Aβ degradation pathway.*

influence on the level of toxicity or fibrillization of amylin [57, 58]. Testosterone may regulate the enzymes NEP and IDE and improve the AD conditions [53]. Another protein, the APOE ε4 allele is very related to the AD, promoting β-amyloid peptides clearance, and it was found that the isoform ApoE ε2 and ApoE ε3 are very efficient than the ApoE ε4 protein. The modification among the isoform may influence the ability of ApoE to promote β-amyloid peptides degradation, and the modification of ApoE is subjected by its lipid carrier molecule ABCA1, whereby higher modification may increases the clearance of β-amyloid peptides [59, 60]. The insulin impairment and the brain function are associated with AD [53]. Brain insulin is very special and mostly originated from endogenous production which is not influenced by the plasma insulin [61]. The mechanism of insulin action in the brain describes the signal transduction via signal cascade pathway. In which first insulin binds to the insulin receptors and then phosphorylation occurs on multiple substrates such as insulin receptor substrate-1 and insulin receptor substrate-II. This phosphorylated substrate activates the downstream signaling pathways and activates the phosphatidylinositol 3-kinase, which is an important modulator for synaptic malleability, education, and remembrance. The activation of phosphatidylinositol 3-kinase subsequently activates Akt which phosphorylates enzymes related to glucose metabolism such as glycogen synthase kinase (GSK) 3β. Then GSK3β regulates tau protein phosphorylation in AD, and thereby leading to neurofibrillary tangle formation [62, 63]. In vitro and in vivo studies demonstrated that impairment of insulin signaling pathway is associated with the AD pathology [64–66]. There is a strong linkage among the hormone testosterone, insulin and glucose metabolism through glucose transporter and insulin receptor protein [67]. Studies have shown that testosterone influence the glucose uptake and transporter via activation of liver kinase B1/AMP-activated protein kinase signaling pathway in fat cell, where AMPK plays an important role for decreasing mTOR signaling activity and promotes lysosomal degradation of β-amyloid peptides in AD. However, this mechanism can also lead to β-amyloid peptides generation and tau phosphorylation [68, 69]. Several studies have shown that both precursor protein (APP) and β-amyloid peptides co-localize in mitochondria, suggesting the possibility of mitochondrial function is associated with APP biology [70]. Ketone bodies may block the mitochondrial amyloid entry and improve understanding capability [71]. This ability would predictably ameliorate Aβ-mediated suppression of respiratory chain function and perhaps could rescue the bioenergetics hypo metabolism that is observed in AD brains [72]. Alternatively, improving mitochondrial performance outright could reduce the production of Aβ and increase the production of soluble APPα [73].

## 5. Dietary pattern for the prevention and treatment of Alzheimer disease

Dietary patterns which are rich in antioxidant and anti-inflammatory properties, may involve the establishment of auspicious attitudes in the treatment of intellectual deterioration or suspending the development of dementia in the brain [74]. The bio ingredient of diet can change the epigenetic by regulating deoxyribonucleic acid (DNA) modification such as methylation, acetylation, histone protein modifications, and changes of gene expression in the ribonucleic acid (RNA) level. The epigenetic modification may influence the expression of particular genes and subsequently particular marker molecules that are responsible for epigenetic alterations [75]. Lipidation of several molecules are important for brain function, one of them are polyunsaturated fatty acids (PUFAs) [76]. The PUFA are the important component of neuronal cell membranes, which is responsible for membrane fluidity. The crossing of molecules through the membrane allows them for cell signaling and neuronal protection [77]. The essential PUFAs play not only neuroprotection but also involve development and brain functions. They also have antioxidant, anti-excitotoxic, and anti-inflammatory activities in the brain. Imbalance of PUFA has been found in neuropsychiatric health including dementia. The beneficial effects of long-chain omega-3 PUFAs have been observed in populations where long-chain omega-3 PUFAs effectively reduce the risk of cerebral damage in individuals without dementia. This is supported by other studies in such a way that omega-3 fatty acid may effectively reduce the initial stages of intellectual deterioration [78]. Another dietary bioactive compound, curcumin (turmeric powder), plays an important role against β-amyloid peptides deposition in the AD because they have potent antioxidant, anti-inflammatory, and neuroprotective function [79]. The bioactive compound, curcumin, regulates the genetic control by down regulation of several gene expression such as class I HDACs (HDAC1, HDAC3, and HDAC8) and enhances the acetylation of histone H4 levels. The curcumin regulates not only gene expression but also can inhibit certain epigenetic enzymes [80]. Other dietary bioactive compounds, flavonoids have potent antioxidant properties, can modulate epigenetic control by the down regulation of pro-inflammatory and inflammatory cytokines and prevent neural impairment in AD [81, 82]. Thus, flavonoids could be a promising therapeutic intervention against neurodegenerative disease. In vivo and in vitro studies showed that the bioactive compound quercetin may regulates cytokines via activation of several downstream molecules such as nuclear factor (Nrf2), Paraoxonase-2, c-Jun N-terminal kinase (c-JNK), Protein kinase C (PKC), Mitogen-activated protein kinase (MAPK) signaling cascades, and PI3K/Akt pathways [83]. Dietary source of component such as cocoa and seed coat of the black soybean, rich source of plant flavonoids and anthocyanin respectively, have been shown neuroprotective action against intellectual deterioration, oxidative stress, neurodegeneration, and memory impairment in a mouse model of AD via the PI3K/Akt/Nrf2/HO-1 pathways [84, 85]. The dietary patterns of coffee and tea that contain bioactive caffeine have been shown to reverse intellectual impairment and reduce the β-amyloid peptides aggregation in the brain in mice model of AD. This reduction occurs due to the stimulation of protein kinase A activity by the caffeine and increases the phospho-CREB levels, subsequently reducing the phospho-JNK and phosphor-ERK expression in the brain. Thus, the high level of blood caffeine may inhibit the progression to dementia [86, 87]. Dietary pattern of grapes and red wine that contains resveratrol, a polyphenol of potent antioxidant and anti-inflammatory actions [88]. The reactive oxygen species (ROS) induced oxidative stress is protected by the resveratrol by the activation of sirtuin 1 (SIRT1) [89]. Resveratrol also activates a transcriptional coactivator of energy metabolism and several studies have shown that resveratrol supplementation with vitamin D could prevent intellectual impairment in vivo through Amyloidogenic pathways [90, 91]. Another study stated that resveratrol may ameliorate the hippocampal neurodegeneration and memory performance [92]. Insufficient dietary minerals may adversely affect the critical cellular processes associated with intellectual impairment and dementia. Thus, dietary patterns of sufficient minerals may have a protective role against many metabolic diseases including intellectual deterioration [93, 94]. Compelling evidence shows that magnesium deficiency may impair memory and contributes to AD pathology [95]. Magnesium sufficient dietary patterns may modify AβPP processing and stimulate the α-secretase cleavage pathway, thereby protecting the cognitive dysfunction [96].

Dietary patterns of vitamin rich food might be useful in maintaining intellectual function and delaying the progression of AD. Studies have stated that vitamin rich dietary patterns such as folic acid and vitamin B12 can significantly improve intellectual functions [97]. In AD, oxidative stress and mitochondrial dysfunction can be prevented by vitamins, because vitamin can modulate the oxidative stress

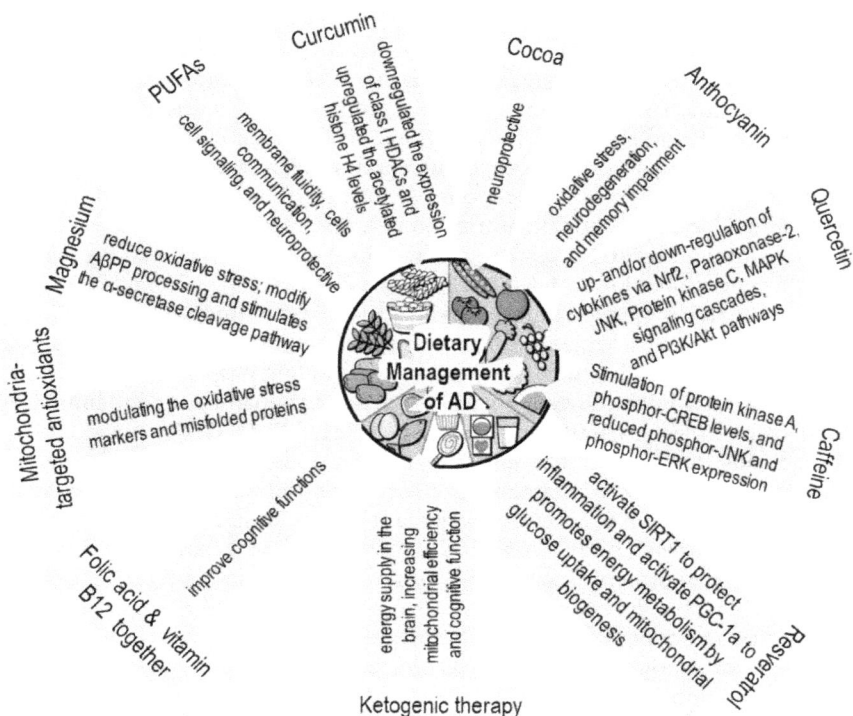

**Figure 4.**
*Mechanism of how dietary patterns are involved for the treatment of AD.*

markers and misfolded proteins [98, 99]. Clinical studies suggested that ketogenic therapies may be beneficial for AD patients. It was found that plasma ketone levels were increased by the medium chain triglyceride and ketone ester supplementa-tions and improved the intellectual function in AD patients [100]. Another source of fuel for the brain is ketone bodies (KB), which may provide energy for the brain and also increase mitochondrial efficiency and cognitive function. The two forms of KB are very important for these mechanisms in the brain; beta-hydroxybutyrate (b-HB) and acetoacetate. Evidence suggests that brain ketone body utilization is not problematic in AD like glucose, making it an alternative energy source of brain function [101]. **Figure 4** summarized the dietary management of AD.

## 6. The mechanism of how exercise-eating patterns can modulate the brain function of AD

In the brain of an AD patient, there are several mechanisms for the changes of β-amyloid peptides synthesis and degradation and tau protein modification. Physical activity may change many signaling molecules both at the mRNA and protein level that may induce the anatomical changes of the brain, chemical and electrophysiological change of the nerve, subsequently enhance the plasticity of neurons of the brain and improve the brain function. Multiple paths of physical exercise and dietary pattern are likely enabled to adjust the level of β-amyloid peptides and tau protein directly or indirectly. Both physical activity and habitu-ated dietary healthy food are effective interventions in such a way that can limit the prevalence of neurodegenerative diseases through the minimization of mitochon-drial dysfunction in bioenergetics processes [102, 103]. Physical exercise play an important role on neuroplasticity of the brain and cellular energy homeostasis well as improve the cognitive functions by controlling the activation of several signaling molecules such as PGC-1α and a nicotinamide adenosine dinucleotide (NAD)-dependent deacetylase, SIRT1 [104, 105]. There is a loss of muscle mass and muscle activity with elderly people. Thus, regular exercise and a healthy dietary pattern reduces the development of aging-related muscle deterioration and promotes muscle activity with the older people [106]. Few have shown the that efficacy of exercise with men and women in AD people, even though differences were found in men and women cognitive improvement with exercise. Study showed that exercise can modulate insulin action and as well as blood glucose [107]. In vivo and clinical study have shown the benefit of exercise and dietary pattern as a non-pharmlogical option in reducing the β-amyloid peptides aggregation and tau protein phosphory-lation in the aging brain. This mechanism happens less in women rather than men due to the change of hormone level [108]. In vivo study stated that exercise and healthy dietary patterns can reduce cortical BACE1 expression and activity by modulating the MAPK signaling in the cortex in AD patients [109].

Interestingly, animal and human studies have shown that exercise and specific dietary patterns may increase testosterone production but it is depending on the intensity of exercise and exercise-induced testosterone sustained for a long time in the body. It was found that high intensity of exercise can increase testosterone levels in T2DM patients, which is important for the reduction of risk factors of AD [110].

The most important neurotrophins, BDNF (brain-derived neurotrophic factor) is responsible for neurogenesis and synaptogenesis. Not only can the central nervous system (CNS) produce the BDNF but also skeletal muscle through the exercise. The underlying molecular mechanisms of exercise to produce testosterone may be medi-ated by BDNF production in the brain. Physical exercise may increase testosterone. Thus, exercise and dietary patterns may increase BDNF levels as a stimulus for the induction of neurogenesis to improve synaptic plasticity [111, 112]. Together physical exercise and dietary patterns not only increase the BDNF but also increase the insulin like growth factor-I (IGF-I). The mechanism of exercise and dietary pattern have been shown to enhance IGF-1 expression in the brain [113]. Moreover, exercise may release several factors like BDNF and IGF-1 into the circulation by testosterone activation. Neurocognitive damage is lifelong incidence with cellular dysfunction. For instance, impairment of BDNF production may influence the synaptic plasticity and neurogenesis in the aging adult brain [114, 115]. Exercise as well as dietary patterns such as low-calorie intake is another important intervention for enlightening metabolic health. The molecular mechanism of low-calorie intake (LCI) is effective against ROS induced-oxidative stress, in which the LCI can reduce β-amyloid peptides aggregation and γ-secretase and plays a preventive role in AD pathology [116, 117]. It was found that the mechanism of low-calorie intake exerts its action by inhibiting nutrient-sensing and inflammatory pathways, thus physical activity and dietary pattern may also be effective methods for the preventive measures of AD [118]. The cellular energy homeostasis is mediated by AMPK in mitochondria, adipose tissue, skeletal muscle, and liver. This mechanism is activated by LKB1 and in response to metabolic stresses, exercise, sex hormones, and insulin sensitizing agents such as Metformin. Thus, the physical exercise and healthy dietary pattern plays a key role in AD patients [119–121]. Oxidative stress and inflammation are the hallmarks of dementia. Individuals' cognitive abilities are related to both non-modifiable factors and modifiable risk factors such as exercise and dietary status. Low calorie diet may be effective against cognitive decline and the high calorie is vice versa [122]. Additionally, some dietary patterns that contain bioactive compounds

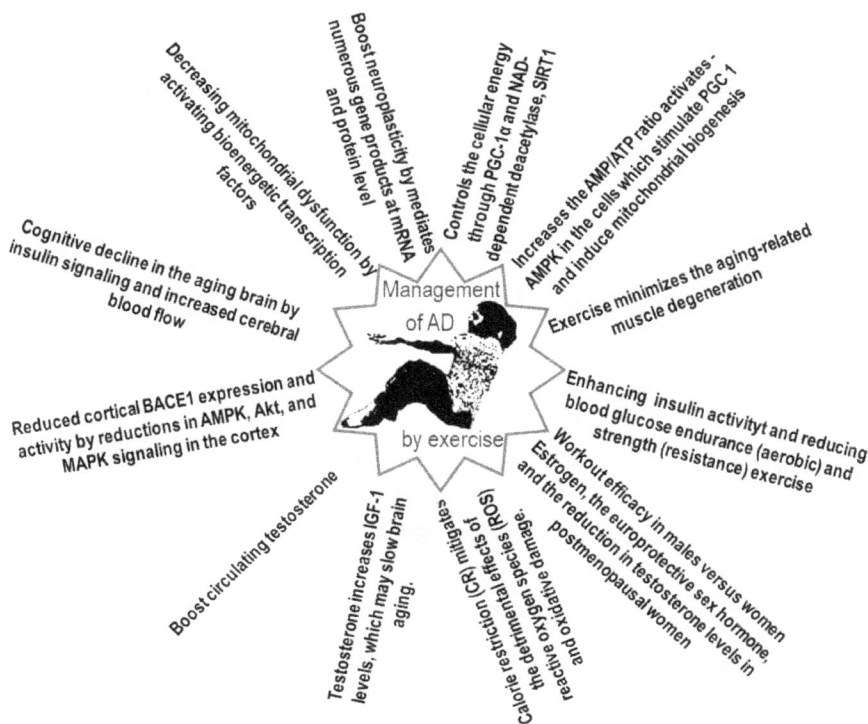

**Figure 5.**
*Mechanism of exercise mediated management of AD.*

may increase signaling molecules and neuronal hormones that are responsible for cognitive improvement. Diet therapy such as vitamin rich food may affect the bodies' central metabolism as well as brain function, and the production of neurotransmitters for modulation of mood in AD [123, 124]. Conversely, it was found that lack of basic B complex (folic acid, B6, and B12) in the dietary pattern is also proposed to impact on the rate of brain atrophy associated with mild cognitive impairment (MCI) [125]. Strength exercise and other dietary patterns such as intake of seafood and other sources of long-chain omega-3 polyunsaturated fats (LC-n3-FA) may have long-term beneficial effects on cognitive function [126, 127]. Thus, exercise and dietary patterns may balance several factors such as LC-n3-FA act via BDNF, and insulin-like growth factor-1 (IGF-1) can alter the expression of a number of protein pathways in neuronal function, plasticity, and neurogenesis [128]. **Figure 5** summarized the exercise and dietary management of AD.

## 7. Social inclusion for the treatment of AD

Social inclusion is multidimensional including social and cultural connection with family, friends, work, personal interests and local community, deal with personal crisis etc., and operates at various social levels. In AD, the deterioration of brain activity begins in the hippocampus areas primarily associated with memory and emotion. The deterioration then spreads to other regions, resulting in reduced neuronal processing, eventually associated with episodic memory, emotion and mood, sensation, self-awareness, attention, memory retrieval and theory of mind which is adversely affected in the early stages of AD. Thus, it could be suggested that the brain regions affected by AD may share something in common, including their role of regulating emotion, memory and awareness and social inclusion can significantly affect in a broad range of measures, including a reduction of cognitive decline, reduction in perceived stress, increase in quality of life, as well as increases in functional connectivity, percent volume brain change and cerebral blood flow in areas of the cortex [129–131]. For the treatment of AD, Social inclusion is potentially beneficial in improving the cognitive function of older adults with mild to moderate dementia and improving their quality of life. Thus, it is recognized as a priority field of AD research, as pharmacologic treatments have not demonstrated effective outcomes [132]. Social inclusion may promote communication and enhance social interaction skills that are important for potentially beneficial cognitive functions and domains of memory and recall of older adults with dementia. These non-pharmacological interventions aim to reduce the behavioral symptoms of the AD. For instance, music therapy involves listening to music and singing songs, can modulate the factors involved in cognition and conduct, divert the attention of older adults to provoke emotional responses and modulate them, draw on different cognitive functions, and evoke movement patterns. Another study has indicated that singing traditional songs, which emerged from the life experiences of people living with dementia, activates their implicit memory with a priming effect [133]. Traditional opera can potentially be an effective therapy for improving the cognitive function of older adults with dementia, reducing their behavioral and psychiatric symptoms and enhancing their quality of life [134]. Moreover, it helps improve their memory as well as the coherence and expressiveness of their speech [135]. About ninety percent people with dementia showed behavioral and psychological symptoms and can cause serious complications but reduction of this complication by use of single antipsychotic medications is very difficult. Several studies showed that consideration of both the physical and the social inclusion can promote self-determination and opportunities for meaning and purpose of persons with dementia [136]. Recent studies concluded that the level of evidence is considered insufficient to support the use of single non pharmacological interventions in prevention efforts of AD; however, mega study reported that around one third of ADs cases worldwide might be attributable to potentially modifiable risk factors such as smoking, physical inactivity, and midlife obesity [137].

## 8. Conclusion

Single nonpharmacological interventions for the treatment of pathophysiological hallmarks of AD was not sufficient. It should include a new approach of three effector modulations such as exercise–eating pattern and social (EES) activities for the treatment of AD. However, when considering the single modulator exercise, adapting the physical environment is necessary but not sufficient. To effectively address AD, the exercise and eating pattern must also be incorporated into the intervention. Also, when considering social inclusion related to initiatives aimed at decreasing AD, providing initial training is necessary, ongoing training and support to mindfulness, meditation in the form of effective enabling and reinforcing factors must also be included. Finally, development of individualized approaches that promote self-control exercise, eating patterns and social inclusion of persons with dementia. This new approach EES should also be included with other interventions aimed at decreasing AD. Though it is very important that the combination of EES and other interventions would be supportive by the success of interventions. It is our hope that this new approach EES also provides direction for future research and initiatives aimed at successful and sustainable nonpharmacological management of AD.

## Acknowledgements

I am particularly grateful Jashore University of Science and Technology for the logistic support of this review article.

Author details

Afroza Sultana and Md Alauddin*
Department of Nutrition and Food Technology, Jashore University of Science and Technology, Bangladesh

*Address all correspondence to: mdalauddin_nft@just.edu.bd

IntechOpen

# References

[1] Alzheimer's Association. 2019 Alzheimer's disease facts and figures. Alzheimer's & Dementia. 2019;**15**: 321-387. DOI: 10.1016/j.jalz. 2019.01.010

[2] Yaghoubi A. The Effects of Aerobic Training and Omega-3 Intake on Aβ42, Neprilysin, and γ- Secretase in the Hippocampus of Male Rats Alzheimer's model. Tehran, Iran: Islamic Azad University; 2021. DOI: 10.21203/ rs.3.rs-427829/v1

[3] Murphy MP, LeVine H. Alzheimer's disease and amyloid-β peptide'. Journal of Alzheimer's disease. 2020;**19**:311. DOI: 10.3233/JAD-2010-1221

[4] Bhatti GK, Reddy AP, Reddy PH, Bhatti JS. Lifestyle modifications and nutritional interventions in aging-associated cognitive decline and Alzheimer's disease. Frontiers in Aging Neuroscience. 2020;**11**:369

[5] Beydoun MA, Beydoun HA, Gamaldo AA, Teel A, Zonderman AB, Wang Y. Epidemiologic studies of modifiable factors associated with cognition and dementia: systematic review and meta-analysis. BMC Public Health. 2014;**14**(1):643

[6] UN Department of Economic and Social Affairs, Population Division. World population ageing 2013 [Internet]. 2013. ST/ESA/SER.A/348. [cited 2016 Jun 24]. Available from: http://www.un.org/esa/socdev/ documents/ageing/Data/World PopulationAgeingReport2013.pdf

[7] Ngandu T, Lehtisalo J, Solomon A, Levalahti E, Ahtiluoto S, Antikainen R, et al. A 2 year multidomain intervention of diet, exercise, cognitive training and vascular risk monitoring versus control to prevent cognitive decline in at-risk elderly people (FINGER): a randomised controlled trial. Lancet. 2015;**385**:2255-2263. DOI: 10.1016/S0140-6736(15)60461-5

[8] Kolarova M, Garcia-Sierra F, Bartos A, Ricny J, Ripova D. Structure and pathology of tau protein in Alzheimer disease. International Journal of Alzheimer's Disease. 2012;**2012**:731526. DOI: 10.1155/2012/731526

[9] Lee VM, Goedert M, Trojanowski JQ. Neurodegenerative tauopathies. Annual Review of Neuroscience. 2001;**24**: 1121-1159

[10] Holmes C, Boche D, Wilkinson D, Yadegarfar G, Hopkins V, Bayer A, et al. Long-term effects of Abeta42 immunization in Alzheimer's disease: follow-up of a randomized, placebo-controlled phase I trial. Lancet. 2008;**372**:216-223

[11] Uslu S, Akarkarasu ZE, Ozbabalik D, Ozkan S, Çolak O, Demirkan ES, et al. Levels of amyloid beta-42, interleukin-6 and tumor necrosis factor-alpha in Alzheimer's disease and vascular dementia. Neurochemical Research. 2012;**37**(7):1554-1559

[12] Capetillo-Zarate E, Gracia L, Tampellini D, Gouras GK. Intraneuronal Aβ accumulation, amyloid plaques, and synapse pathology in Alzheimer's disease. Neurodegenerative Diseases. 2012;**10**(1-4):56-59

[13] Cavallucci V, D'Amelio M, Cecconi F. Aβ toxicity in Alzheimer's disease. Molecular Neurobiology. 2012;**45**(2):366-378

[14] Mosconi L. Brain glucose metabolism in the early and specific diagnosis of Alzheimer's disease: FDG-PET studies in MCI and AD. European Journal of Nuclear Medicine and Molecular Imaging. 2005;**32**: 486-510

[15] Smith AD, Smith SM, De Jager CA, Whitbread P, Johnston C, Agacinski G, et al. Homocysteine lowering by B vitamins slows the rate of accelerated brain atrophy in mild cognitive impairment: a randomized controlled trial. PLoS One. 2010;**5**(9):e12244

[16] Obeid R, Herrmann W. Mechanisms of homocysteine neurotoxicity in neurodegenerative diseases with special reference to dementia. FEBS Letters. 2006;**580**(13):2994-3005

[17] Kamat P, Vacek J, Kalani A, Tyagi N. Homocysteine induced cerebrovascular dysfunction: a link to Alzheimer's disease etiology. The Open Neurology Journal. 2015;**9**:9

[18] Pi T, Liu B, Shi J. Abnormal homocysteine metabolism: An insight of Alzheimer's disease from DNA methylation. Behavioral Neurology. 2020;**2020**:11. Article ID: 8438602

[19] Tawfik A, Mohamed R, Kira D, Alhusban S, Al-Shabrawey M. N-Methyl-D-aspartate receptor activation, novel mechanism of homocysteine-induced blood–retinal barrier dysfunction. Journal of Molecular Medicine. 2021;**99**(1):119-130

[20] Selkoe DJ. Alzheimer's disease: genes, proteins, and therapy. Physiological Reviews. 2001;**81**:741-766

[21] Dislich B, Lichtenthaler SF. The membrane-bound aspartyl protease BACE1: Molecular and functional properties in Alzheimer's disease and beyond. Frontiers in Physiology. 2012;**3**:8

[22] Cole SL, Vassar R. The basic biology of BACE1: A key therapeutic target for Alzheimer's disease. Current Genomics. 2007;**8**:509-530

[23] Dominguez D, Tournoy J, Hartmann D, Huth T, Cryns K, Deforce S, et al. Phenotypic and biochemical analyses of BACE1- and BACE2-deficient mice. The Journal of Biological Chemistry. 2005;**280**: 30797-30806

[24] Schechter I, Ziv E. Kinetic properties of cathepsin D and BACE 1 indicate the need to search for additional beta-secretase candidate(s). Biological Chemistry. 2008;**389**:313-320

[25] Samaan MC, Anand SS, Sharma AM, Samjoo IA, Tarnopolsky MA. Sex differences in skeletal muscle phosphatase and tensin homolog deleted on chromosome 10 (PTEN) levels: A cross-sectional study. Scientific Reports. 2015;**5**:9154

[26] Hoffmeister A, Tuennemann J, Sommerer I, Mossner J, Rittger A, Schleinitz D, et al. Genetic and biochemical evidence for a functional role of BACE1 in the regulation of insulin mRNA expression. Obesity (Silver Spring). 2013;**21**:E626-E633

[27] Uchoa MF, Moser VA, Pike CJ. Interactions between inflammation, sex steroids, and Alzheimer's disease risk factors. Frontiers in Neuroendocrinology. 2016;**43**:60-82

[28] Kristiansen OP, Mandrup-Poulsen T. Interleukin-6 and diabetes: The good, the bad, or the indifferent? Diabetes. 2005;**54**(2):S114-S124

[29] Rubio-Perez JM, Morillas-Ruiz JM. A review: Inflammatory process in Alzheimer's disease, role of cytokines. Scientific World Journal. 2012; **2012**:756357

[30] Folli F, Corradi D, Fanti P, Davalli A, Paez A, Giaccari A, et al. The role of oxidative stress in the pathogenesis of type 2 diabetes mellitus micro- and macrovascular complications: Avenues for a mechanistic- based therapeutic approach. Current Diabetes Reviews. 2011;**7**:313-324

[31] Ota H, Akishita M, Akiyoshi T, Kahyo T, Setou M, Ogawa S, et al. Testosterone deficiency accelerates neuronal and vascular aging of SAMP8 mice: Protective role of eNOS and SIRT1. PLoS One. 2012;7:e29598

[32] Cao X, Sudhof TC. A transcriptively active complex of APP with Fe65 and histone acetyltransferase Tip60. Science. 2001;293:115-120

[33] Gao Y, Pimplikar SW. The gamma-secretase-cleaved C-terminal fragment of amyloid precursor protein mediates signaling to the nucleus. Proceedings of the National Academy of Sciences of the United States of America. 2001;98: 14979-14984

[34] Kimberly WT, Zheng JB, Guenette SY, Selkoe DJ. The intracellular domain of the beta-amyloid precursor protein is stabilized by Fe65 and translocates to the nucleus in a notch-like manner. The Journal of Biological Chemistry. 2001;276:40288-40292

[35] Hardy J, Selkoe DJ. The amyloid hypothesis of Alzheimer's disease: progress and problems on the road to therapeutics. Science. 2002;297:353-356

[36] Miller BC, Eckman EA, Sambamurti K, Dobbs N, Chow KM, Eckman CB, et al. Amyloid-beta peptide levels in brain are inversely correlated with insulysin activity levels in vivo. Proceedings of the National Academy of Sciences of the United States of America. 2003;100:6221-6226

[37] Huang SM, Mouri A, Kokubo H, Nakajima R, Suemoto T, Higuchi M, et al. Neprilysin-sensitive synapse-associated amyloidbeta peptide oligomers impair neuronal plasticity and cognitive function. The Journal of Biological Chemistry. 2006;281: 17941-17951

[38] Qiu WQ, Folstein MF. Insulin, insulin-degrading enzyme and amyloid-beta peptide in Alzheimer's disease: review and hypothesis. Neurobiology of Aging. 2006;27:190-198

[39] Luchsinger JA, Tang MX, Shea S, Mayeux R. Hyperinsulinemia and risk of Alzheimer disease. Neurology. 2004;63:1187-1192

[40] Sun B, Zhou Y, Halabisky B, Lo I, Cho SH, Mueller-Steiner S, et al. Cystatin C-cathepsin B axis regulates amyloid beta levels and associated neuronal deficits in an animal model of Alzheimer's disease. Neuron. 2008;60:247-257

[41] Grimm MO, Mett J, Stahlmann CP, Haupenthal VJ, Zimmer VC, Hartmann T. Neprilysin and Aβ clearance: impact of the APP intracellular domain in NEP regulation and implications in Alzheimer's disease. Frontiers in Aging Neuroscience. 2013;5:27. Article 98

[42] Shibata M, Yamada S, Kumar SR, Calero M, Bading J, Frangione B, et al. Clearance of Alzheimer's amyloid-ss(1-40) peptide from brain by LDL receptor-related protein-1 at the blood-brain barrier. The Journal of Clinical Investigation. 2000;106:1489-1499

[43] Deane R, Du Yan S, Submamaryan RK, LaRue B, Jovanovic S, Hogg E, et al. RAGE mediates amyloid-beta peptide transport across the blood-brain barrier and accumulation in brain. Nature Medicine. 2003;9:907-913

[44] Zlokovic BV. Neurovascular mechanisms of Alzheimer's neuro-degeneration. Trends in Neurosciences. 2005;28:202-208

[45] Mielke MM, Vemuri P, Rocca WA. Clinical epidemiology of Alzheimer's disease: Assessing sex and gender differences. Clinical Epidemiology. 2014;6:37-48

[46] Gandy S, Almeida OP, Fonte J, Lim D, Waterrus A, Spry N, et al. Chemical andropause and amyloid-beta peptide. JAMA. 2001;**285**:2195-2196

[47] Schulz K, Korz V. Hippocampal testosterone relates to reference memory performance and synaptic plasticity in male rats. Frontiers in Behavioral Neuroscience. 2010;**4**:187

[48] Jia JX, Cui CL, Yan XS, Zhang BF, Song W, Huo DS, et al. Effects of testosterone on synaptic plasticity mediated by androgen receptors in male SAMP8 mice. Journal of Toxicology and Environmental Health. Part A. 2016;**79**:849-855

[49] Atwi S, McMahon D, Scharfman H, MacLusky NJ. Androgen modulation of hippocampal structure and function. The Neuroscientist. 2016;**22**:46-60

[50] Rosario ER, Pike CJ. Androgen regulation of betaamyloid protein and the risk of Alzheimer's disease. Brain Research Reviews. 2008;**57**:444-453

[51] Rosario ER, Carroll J, Pike CJ. Testosterone regulation of Alzheimer-like neuropathology in male 3xTg-AD mice involves both estrogen and androgen pathways. Brain Research. 2010;**1359**:281-290

[52] Papalia MA, Davis SR. What is the rationale for androgen therapy for women? Treatments in Endocrinology. 2003;**2**:77-84

[53] Asih PR, Tegg ML, Sohrabi H, Carruthers M, Gandy SE, Saad F, et al. Multiple mechanisms linking type 2 diabetes and Alzheimer's disease: testosterone as a modifier. Journal of Alzheimer's Disease. 2017;**59**(2):445-466. DOI: 10.3233/JAD-161259

[54] McAllister C, Long J, Bowers A, Walker A, Cao P, Honda S, et al. Genetic targeting aromatase in male amyloid precursor protein transgenic mice down-regulates beta-secretase (BACE1) and prevents Alzheimer-like pathology and cognitive impairment. The Journal of Neuroscience. 2010;**30**:7326-7334

[55] Vieira JS, Saraiva KL, Barbosa MC, Porto RC, Cresto JC, Peixoto CA, et al. Effect of dexamethasone and testosterone treatment on the regulation of insulin-degrading enzyme and cellular changes in ventral rat prostate after castration. International Journal of Experimental Pathology. 2011;**92**:272-280

[56] Yao M, Nguyen TV, Rosario ER, Ramsden M, Pike CJ. Androgens regulate neprilysin expression: Role in reducing beta-amyloid levels. Journal of Neurochemistry. 2008;**105**:2477-2488

[57] Bennett RG, Duckworth WC, Hamel FG. Degradation of amylin by insulin-degrading enzyme. The Journal of Biological Chemistry. 2000;**275**: 36621-36625

[58] Guan H, Chow KM, Shah R, Rhodes CJ, Hersh LB. Degradation of islet amyloid polypeptide by neprilysin. Diabetologia. 2012;**55**:2989-2998

[59] Verghese PB, Castellano JM, Garai K, Wang Y, Jiang H, Shah A, et al. ApoE influences amyloid-beta (Abeta) clearance despite minimal apoE/Abeta association in physiological conditions. Proceedings of the National Academy of Sciences of the USA. 2013;**110**: E1807-E1816

[60] Wildsmith KR, Holley M, Savage JC, Skerrett R, Landreth GE. Evidence for impaired amyloid beta clearance in Alzheimer's disease. Alzheimer's Research & Therapy. 2013;**5**:33

[61] Blazquez E, Velazquez E, Hurtado-Carneiro V, Ruiz-Albusac JM. Insulin in the brain: Its pathophysiological implications for States related with central insulin resistance, type 2 diabetes and

Alzheimer's disease. Front Endocrinol (Lausanne). 2014;**5**:161

[62] Hooper C, Killick R, Lovestone S. The GSK3 hypothesis of Alzheimer's disease. Journal of Neurochemistry. 2008;**104**:1433-1439

[63] Rayasam GV, Tulasi VK, Sodhi R, Davis JA, Ray A. Glycogen synthase kinase 3: More than a namesake. British Journal of Pharmacology. 2009; **156**:885-898

[64] Yang Y, Ma D, Wang Y, Jiang T, Hu S, Zhang M, et al. Intranasal insulin ameliorates tau hyperphosphorylation in a rat model of type 2 diabetes. Journal of Alzheimer's Disease. 2013;**33**:329-338

[65] Verdile G, Keane KN, Cruzat VF, Medic S, Sabale M, Rowles J, et al. Inflammation and oxidative stress: The molecular connectivity between insulin resistance, obesity, and Alzheimer's disease. Mediators of Inflammation. 2015;**2015**:105828

[66] Verdile G, Fuller SJ, Martins RN. The role of type 2 diabetes in neurodegeneration. Neurobiology of Disease. 2015;**84**:22-38

[67] Rao PM, Kelly DM, Jones TH. Testosterone and insulin resistance in the metabolic syndrome and T2DM in men. Nature Reviews. Endocrinology. 2013;**9**:479-493

[68] Mitsuhashi K, Senmaru T, Fukuda T, Yamazaki M, Shinomiya K, Ueno M, et al. Testosterone stimulates glucose uptake and GLUT4 translocation through LKB1/AMPK signaling in 3T3-L1 adipocytes. Endocrine. 2016;**51**:174-184

[69] Cai Z, Yan LJ, Li K, Quazi SH, Zhao B. Roles of AMP-activated protein kinase in Alzheimer's disease. Neuromolecular Medicine. 2012;**14**:1-14

[70] Devi L, Prabhu BM, Galati DF, Avadhani NG, Anandatheerthavarada HK. Accumulation of amyloid precursor protein in the mitochondrial import channels of human Alzheimer's disease brain is associated with mitochondrial dysfunction. The Journal of Neuroscience. 2006;**26**:9057-9068

[71] Yin JX, Maalouf M, Han P, Zhao M, Gao M, Dharshaun T, et al. Ketones block amyloid entry and improve cognition in an Alzheimer's model. Neurobiology of Aging. 2016;**39**:25-37

[72] Swerdlow RH. Mitochondria and cell bioenergetics: increasingly recognized components and a possible etiologic cause of Alzheimer's disease. Antioxidants & Redox Signaling. 2012c;**16**:1434-1455

[73] Hasebe N, Fujita Y, Ueno M, Yoshimura K, Fujino Y, Yamashita T. Soluble beta-amyloid Precursor Protein Alpha binds to p75 neurotrophin receptor to promote neurite outgrowth. PLoS One. 2013;**8**:e82321

[74] Canevelli M, Lucchini F, Quarata F, Bruno G, Cesari M. Nutrition and dementia: evidence for preventive approaches? Nutrients. 2016;**8**:144. DOI: 10.3390/nu8030144

[75] Abdul QA, Yu BP, Chung HY, Jung HA, Choi JS. Epigenetic modifications of gene expression by lifestyle and environment. Archives of Pharmacal Research. 2017;**40**:1219-1237. DOI: 10.1007/s12272-017-0973-3

[76] Bazan NG. Lipid signaling in neural plasticity, brain repair, and neuroprotection. Molecular Neurobiology. 2005;**32**:89-103. DOI: 10.1385/mn:32:1:089

[77] Liu JJ, Green P, John Mann J, Rapoport SI, Sublette ME. Pathways of polyunsaturated fatty acid utilization: implications for brain function in neuropsychiatric health and disease. Brain Research. 2015;**1597**:220-246. DOI: 10.1016/j.brainres.2014.11.059

[78] Thomas J, Thomas CJ, Radcliffe J, Itsiopoulos C. Omega-3 fatty acids in early prevention of inflammatory neurodegenerative disease: a focus on Alzheimer's disease. BioMed Research International. 2015;**2015**:172801. DOI: 10.1155/2015/172801

[79] Reddy PH, Manczak M, Yin X, Grady MC, Mitchell A, Tonk S, et al. Protective effects of Indian spice curcumin against amyloid-b in Alzheimer's disease. Journal of Alzheimer's Disease. 2018;**61**:843-866. DOI: 10.3233/JAD-170512

[80] Vahid F, Zand H, Nosrat-Mirshekarlou E, Najafi R, Hekmatdoost A. The role dietary of bioactive compounds on the regulation of histone acetylases and deacetylases: a review. Gene. 2015;**562**:8-15. DOI: 10.1016/j.gene.2015.02.045

[81] Fernandes I, Pérez-Gregorio R, Soares S, Mateus N, De Freitas V. Wine flavonoids in health and disease prevention. Molecules. 2017;**22**:E292. DOI: 10.3390/molecules22020292

[82] Spagnuolo C, Moccia S, Russo GL. Anti-inflammatory effects of flavonoids in neurodegenerative disorders. European Journal of Medicinal Chemistry. 2018;**153**:105-115. DOI: 10.1016/j.ejmech.2017.09.001

[83] Zaplatic E, Bule M, Shah SZA, Uddin MS, Niaz K. Molecular mechanisms underlying protective role of quercetin in attenuating Alzheimer's disease. Life Sciences. 2019;**224**:109-119. DOI: 10.1016/j.lfs.2019.03.055

[84] Lamport DJ, Pal D, Moutsiana C, Field DT, Williams CM, Spencer JP, et al. The effect of flavanol-rich cocoa on cerebral perfusion in healthy older adults during conscious resting state: a placebo controlled, crossover, acute trial. Psychopharmacology. 2015;**232**:3227-3234. DOI: 10.1007/s00213-015-3972-4

[85] Ali T, Kim T, Rehman SU, Khan MS, Amin FU, Khan M, et al. Natural dietary supplementation of anthocyanins via PI3K/Akt/Nrf2/HO-1 pathways mitigate oxidative stress, neurodegeneration, and memory impairment in a mouse model of Alzheimer's disease. Molecular Neurobiology. 2018;**55**:6076-6093. DOI: 10.1007/s12035-017-0798-6

[86] Zeitlin R, Patel S, Burgess S, Arendash GW, Echeverria V. Caffeine induces beneficial changes in PKA signaling and JNK and ERK activities in the striatum and cortex of Alzheimer's transgenic mice. Brain Research. 2011;**1417**:127-136. DOI: 10.1016/j.brainres.2011.08.036

[87] Cao C, Loewenstein DA, Lin X, Zhang C, Wang L, Duara R, et al. High blood caffeine levels in MCI linked to lack of progression to dementia. Journal of Alzheimer's Disease. 2012;**30**:559-572. DOI: 10.3233/jad-2012-111781

[88] Sawda C, Moussa C, Turner RS. Resveratrol for Alzheimer's disease. Annals of the New York Academy of Sciences. 2017;**1403**:142-149. DOI: 10.1111/nyas.13431

[89] Cantó C, Gerhart-Hines Z, Feige JN, Lagouge M, Noriega L, Milne JC, et al. AMPK regulates energy expenditure by modulating NADC metabolism and SIRT1 activity. Nature. 2009;**458**:1056-1060. DOI: 10.1038/nature07813

[90] Cheng J, Rui Y, Qin L, Xu J, Han S, Yuan L, et al. Vitamin D combined with resveratrol prevents cognitive decline in SAMP8 mice. Current Alzheimer Research. 2017;**14**:820-833. DOI: 10.2174/1567205014666170207093455

[91] Izquierdo V, Palomera-Ávalos V, López-Ruiz S, Canudas A-M, Pallàs M, Griñán-Ferré C. Maternal resveratrol supplementation prevents cognitive decline in senescent mice offspring. International Journal of Molecular Sciences. 2019;**20**:E1134. DOI: 10.3390/ijms20051134

[92] Gomes BAQ, Silva JPB, Romeiro CFR, Dos Santos SM, Rodrigues CA, Gonçalves PR, et al. Neuroprotective mechanisms of resveratrol in Alzheimer's disease: role of SIRT1. Oxidative Medicine and Cellular Longevity. 2018;**2018**:8152373. DOI: 10.1155/2018/8152373

[93] Ozawa M, Ninomiya T, Ohara T, Hirakawa Y, Doi Y, Hata J, et al. Self-reported dietary intake of potassium, calcium, and magnesium and risk of dementia in the Japanese: The Hisayama study. Journal of the American Geriatrics Society. 2012;**60**:1515-1520. DOI: 10.1111/j.1532-5415.2012.04061.x

[94] Barbagallo M, Belvedere M, Di Bella G, Dominguez LJ. Altered ionized magnesium levels in mild-to-moderate Alzheimer's disease. Magnesium Research. 2011;**24**:S115-S121. DOI: 10.1684/mrh.2011.0287

[95] Vural H, Demirin H, Kara Y, Eren I, Delibas N. Alterations of plasma magnesium, copper, zinc, iron and selenium concentrations and some related erythrocyte antioxidant enzyme activities in patients with Alzheimer's disease. Journal of Trace Elements in Medicine and Biology. 2010;**24**:169-173. DOI: 10.1016/j.jtemb.2010.02.002

[96] Yu J, Sun M, Chen Z, Lu J, Liu Y, Zhou L, et al. Magnesium modulates amyloid-b protein precursor trafficking and processing. Journal of Alzheimer's Disease. 2010;**20**:1091-1106. DOI: 10.3233/JAD-2010-091444

[97] McCleery J, Abraham RP, Denton DA, Rutjes AW, Chong LY, Al-Assaf AS, et al. Vitamin and mineral supplementation for preventing dementia or delaying cognitive decline in people with mild cognitive impairment. Cochrane Database of Systematic Reviews. 2018; **11**:CD011905. DOI: 10.1002/14651858.cd011905

[98] Manczak M, Mao P, Calkins MJ, Cornea A, Reddy AP, Murphy MP, et al. Mitochondria-targeted antioxidants protect against amyloid-b toxicity in Alzheimer's disease neurons. Journal of Alzheimer's Disease. 2010;**20**: S609-S631. DOI: 10.3233/jad-2010-100564

[99] Reddy PH, Reddy TP. Mitochondria as a therapeutic target for aging and neurodegenerative diseases. Current Alzheimer Research. 2011;**8**:393-409. DOI: 10.2174/156720511795745401

[100] Newport MT, VanItallie TB, Kashiwaya Y, King MT, Veech RL. A new way to produce hyperketonemia: use of ketone ester in a case of Alzheimer's disease. Alzheimer's & Dementia. 2015;**11**:99-103

[101] Broom GM, Shaw IC, Rucklidge JJ. The ketogenic diet as a potential treatment and prevention strategy for Alzheimer's disease. Nutrition. Apr. 1 2019;**60**:118-121

[102] Cotman CW, Berchtold NC. Exercise: a behavioral intervention to enhance brain health and plasticity. Trends in Neurosciences. 2002;**25**(6):295-301

[103] Barbieri E, Agostini D, Polidori E, Potenza L, Guescini M, Lucertini F, et al. The pleiotropic effect of physical exercise on mitochondrial dynamics in aging skeletal muscle. Oxidative Medicine and Cellular Longevity. 2015;**2015**:917085. DOI: 10.1155/2015/917085

[104] Rodgers JT, Lerin C, Haas W, Gygi SP, Spiegelman BM, Puigserver P. Nutrient control of glucose homeostasis through a complex of PGC-1a and SIRT1. Nature. 2005;**434**:113-118. DOI: 10.1038/nature03354

[105] Jäger S, Handschin C, St-Pierre J, Spiegelman BM. AMP-activated protein kinase (AMPK) action in skeletal muscle via direct phosphorylation of PGC-1a. Proceedings of the National Academy of

Sciences of the USA. 2007;**104**:12017-12022. DOI: 10.1073/pnas. 0705070104

[106] Cartee GD, Hepple RT, Bamman MM, Zierath JR. Exercise promotes healthy aging of skeletal muscle. Cell Metabolism. 2016;**23**:1034-1047. DOI: 10.1016/j.cmet.2016.05.007

[107] Balsamo S, Willardson JM, Frederico Sde S, Prestes J, Balsamo DC, da CN D, et al. Effectiveness of exercise on cognitive impairment and Alzheimer's disease. International Journal of General Medicine. 2013;**6**:387-391

[108] Ryan SM, Kelly AM. Exercise as a pro-cognitive, pro-neurogenic and anti-inflammatory intervention in transgenic mouse models of Alzheimer's disease. Ageing Research Reviews. 2016;**27**:77-92

[109] MacPherson RE, Baumeister P, Peppler WT, Wright DC. Little JP (2015) Reduced cortical BACE1 content with one bout of exercise is accompanied by declines in AMPK, Akt, and MAPK signaling in obese, glucose-intolerant mice. Journal of Applied Physiology. 1985;**119**:1097-1104

[110] Bertram S, Brixius K, Brinkmann C. Exercise for the diabetic brain: How physical training may help prevent dementia and Alzheimer's disease in T2DM patients. Endocrine. 2016;**53**:350-363

[111] Verhovshek T, Sengelaub DR. Androgen action at the target musculature regulates brain-derived neurotrophic factor protein in the spinal nucleus of the bulbocavernosus. Developmental Neurobiology. 2013;**73**:587-598

[112] Huang T, Larsen KT, Ried-Larsen M, Moller NC, Andersen LB. The effects of physical activity and exercise on brain-derived

neurotrophic factor in healthy humans: A review. Scandinavian Journal of Medicine & Science in Sports. 2014;**24**:1-10

[113] Allan CA. Sex steroids and glucose metabolism. Asian Journal of Andrology. 2014;**16**:232-238

[114] Peters R. Ageing and the brain. Postgraduate Medical Journal. 2006;**82**:84-88. DOI: 10.1136/pgmj.2005.036665

[115] Mattson MP, Maudsley S, Martin B. BDNF and 5-HT: a dynamic duo in age-related neuronal plasticity and neurodegenerative disorders. Trends in Neurosciences. 2004;**27**(10):589-594. DOI: 10.1016/j.tins.2004.08.001

[116] Wahl D, Solon-Biet SM, Cogger VC, Fontana L, Simpson SJ, Le Couteur DG, et al. Aging, lifestyle and dementia. Neurobiology of Disease. Oct 1 2019;**130**:104481. DOI: 10.1016/j.nbd.2019.104481

[117] Schafer MJ, Alldred MJ, Lee SH, Calhoun ME, Petkova E, Mathews PM, et al. Reduction of b-amyloid and g-secretase by calorie restriction in female Tg2576 mice. Neurobiology of Aging. 2015;**36**:1293-1302. DOI: 10.1016/j.neurobiolaging.2014.10.043

[118] Most J, Tosti V, Redman LM, Fontana L. Calorie restriction in humans: an update. Ageing Research Reviews. 2017;**39**:36-45. DOI: 10.1016/j.arr.2016.08.005

[119] Yamada E, Lee TW, Pessin JE, Bastie CC. Targeted therapies of the LKB1/AMPK pathway for the treatment of insulin resistance. Future Medicinal Chemistry. 2010;**2**:1785-1796

[120] Cai Z, Yan LJ, Li K, Quazi SH, Zhao B. Roles of AMP-activated protein kinase in Alzheimer's disease. Neuromolecular Medicine. 2012;**14**:1-14

[121] McInnes KJ, Brown KA, Hunger NI, Simpson ER. Regulation of LKB1 expression by sex hormones in adipocytes. International Journal of Obesity, (London). 2012;**36**:982-985

[122] Dauncey MJ. Nutrition, the brain and cognitive decline: insights from epi-genetics. European Journal of Clinical Nutrition. 2014;**68**(11):1179-1185. DOI: 10.1038/ejcn.2014.173

[123] Morris MC. Symposium 1: vitamins and cognitive development and performance nutritional determinants of cognitive aging and dementia. The Proceedings of the Nutrition Society. 2012;**71**(1):1-13. DOI: 10.1017/s0029665111003296

[124] Morley JE. Cognition and nutrition. Current Opinion in Clinical Nutrition and Metabolic Care. 2014;**17**(1):1-4. DOI: 10.1097/MCO.0000000000000005

[125] Mathers JC. Nutrition and ageing: knowledge, gaps and research priorities. The Proceedings of the Nutrition Society. 2013;**72**(2):246-250. DOI: 10.1017/s0029665112003023

[126] Gomez-Pinilla F. Brain foods: the effects of nutrients on brain function. Nature Reviews. Neuroscience. 2008;**9**(7):568-578. DOI: 10.1038/nrn2421

[127] Witte VA, Kerti L, Hermannstaedter HM, Fiebach JB, Schuchardt JP, Hahn A, et al. Effects of Omega-3 supplementation on brain structure and function in healthy elderly subjects. Journal of Psychophysiology. 2013;**27**:45-45

[128] Gomez-Pinilla F. The influences of diet and exercise on mental health through hormesis. Ageing Research Reviews. 2008;**7**(1):49-62. DOI: 10.1016/j.arr.2007.04.003

[129] Wagner AD, Shannon BJ, Kahn I, Buckner RL. Parietal lobe contributions to episodic memory retrieval. Trends in Cognitive Sciences. 2005;**9**:445-453

[130] Sorg C, Riedl V, Muhlau M, Calhoun VD, Eichele T, Laer L, et al. Selective changes of resting-state networks in individuals at risk for Alzheimer's disease. Proceedings of the National Academy of Sciences of the USA. 2007;**104**:18760-18765

[131] Russell-Williams J, Jaroudi W, Perich T, Hoscheidt S, El Haj M, Moustafa AA. Mindfulness and meditation: treating cognitive impairment and reducing stress in dementia. Reviews in the Neurosciences. 2018;**29**(7):791-804

[132] Adrienne F. Fathoming the constellations: ways of working with families in music therapy for people with advanced dementia. British Journal of Music Therapy. 2017;**31**:43-49. https://doi.org/. DOI: 10.1177/1359457517691052

[133] Yan C, Mingxian G, Fanfan L. Application of two music intervention modes for patients. Chinese Nursing Research. 2011;**25**:2573-2575. DOI: 10.3969/j. issn.1009-6493.2011.28.014

[134] Chen X, Li D, Xu H, Hu Z. Effect of traditional opera on older adults with dementia. Geriatric Nursing. 2020;**41**(2):118-123

[135] Lee YU. The Effects of the Korean Folk song centered Music Therapy on the Cognitive Function of the Elderly with Alzheimer's Dementia. Unpublished master's thesis. Busan: Church Music Kosin University; 2012

[136] Caspar S, Davis ED, Douziech A, Scott DR. Nonpharmacological management of behavioral and psychological symptoms of dementia:

what works, in what circumstances, and why? Innovation in Aging. 2017; **1**(3):igy001

[137] Friedman DB, Becofsky K, Anderson LA, Bryant LL, Hunter RH, Ivey SL, et al. Public perceptions about risk and protective factors for cognitive health and impairment: a review of the literature. International Psychogeriatrics. 2015;**27**(8):1263-1275